BELIEVE YOU CAN

SUCCEED

TRUE STORIES TO INSPIRE
WOMEN IN BUSINESS

Compiled & Edited
by
SUE WILLIAMS

ACKNOWLEDGEMENTS

This book is truly a team effort. It demonstrates the power of connection, creativity, collaboration and contribution at their best. These important qualities underpin the paradigm shift that is currently taking place in our world and in business.

The intention of the authors is to share the insights gleaned from their own journeys to demonstrate the powerful transformations that occur when we are able to believe. To believe that we are here for a purpose, and that we have all of the inner resources we need to succeed in business and in life. I thank all of the contributors for demonstrating that miracles happen when we realise the power that comes from believing in our own unique gifts and talents.

Sincere thanks go to all those who have contributed, supported and encouraged me in bringing this project to fruition. Thank you for believing in me, as I believe in you!

The deepest gratitude goes to each author and poet who has contributed to this book.

Sue Williams

PRAISE FOR THIS BOOK

"This is a great book - thanks so much Sue for believing and publishing, you are a star. I was only a chapter and a half in when inspiration struck me from its pages. I would recommend this book to everyone male or female; entrepreneur or not, it is a book with heart and soul and will touch and inspire many people" ~ *Louise Walters*

"Sue has a unique style of combining authenticity with a rich rawness enveloped in poetry. Believe! is so emotionally rich. Each contribution from a wide range of perspectives encourages the reader to look deep within our hearts and to connect with our true essence. The result is a luxuriant tapestry encouraging the reader to experience:

Beauty	Inspiration	Empathy"
Enlightenment	Energy	
Love	Verse	

~ *Paramjit Oberoi*

"This is a beautifully written book; the stories are amazing. It filled me with real hope for mankind. I am not an entrepreneur and do not aspire to be but love to have my thoughts filled with positivity, creativity, inspiration and success and this book certainly did the job. Had a few tears occasionally and some smiles, it's a lovely balance of happiness and reality. Recommend buy for all those searching for something uplifting and inspirational" ~ *Jo C*

"What I love about this book is that you get both real-life stories and real-life advice, from real women! It is a gorgeous portfolio of stories that build together to uplift and inspire. I would recommend it for any woman - not just entrepreneurs!" ~ *Sandra Peachey* ~ *Author of Peachey Letters. Love Letters to Life.*

"For me, Sue's book has something for all...I dare you not to find something that resonates with you! I am so looking forward to the paperback... it's the sort of read that I know I will keep going back to!!" ~ *Estelle Lloyd-Thurman* ~ *Tender Loving Care Group*

"Sue's creation of the compelling Believe poem initiated this brilliant book which is filled with inspirational stories, poems and exercises. Through sharing the contributors' moving experiences and learning from their reflections, I've finished the book feeling more self-confident and motivated to achieve my dreams. Thank you, Sue for helping us to Believe!" ~ *Susan Brookes-Morris, Writer and Journalist.*

"This book offers a delightful collection of short stories and poems. Inspirational insights are offered to entrepreneurs and individuals seeking change. Each story provides lessons we can learn from others. The contributors share their secrets on how they found their life purpose. If you're ready to come out of comfort zone and make a difference, this is for you!" ~ *Vanessa Augustus, Motivational Business & Lifestyle Coach*

FOREWORD

We all face change at various stages of life. Personal change, business change, career change. And, as I get older, it seems there is more change in my life rather than less. And when we face change and when we feel stuck, it can be very hard to see our way through. Most of us want to be able to see an end point. To plan for it.

But really, what we most need at those times is a little inspiration. Something that brings a little joy and light and connection to help move us forward. Or at least, to set us in motion.

I am a great believer of the fact that, when you are in motion, great things happen. Whether it's going for a walk, or writing a poem, or connecting with a friend. You'll get ideas, you'll be inspired and you'll simply feel better physically. But why am I telling you this?

Because what Sue has provided in this book is all of that. She's very graciously, and with a large dose of fun, brought together a collection of poems and pieces that she has developed and that she has commissioned from people she's met on her journey.

If you are in need of a little dose of lightness, a little lifting of spirits, then you will find it in this book. One of the contributor's quotes Marianne Williamson in her chapter *"And as we let our own light shine, we unconsciously give other people permission to do the same."*

Let this book shed a little light into your world today.

Cathy Presland - Leadership Coach
https://cathypresland.com

CONTENTS

BELIEVE IN YOUR DREAMS, YOUR LEGACY, YOUR POWER!

Do you often feel disheartened? Does it seem an increasing struggle to start or make a success of your business - as if there are so many different aspects to juggle, and you are the only one desperately trying to keep all those disparate plates spinning safely in the air?

What if you become tired or distracted and let one slip – would they all come crashing down around you, shattering your last ounce of confidence along with the jagged smithereens littering the newly polished floor?

If you relate to this nerve-jangling scenario, you are certainly not alone! I have compiled this anthology on the topic of self-belief to showcase uplifting stories by entrepreneurial and business women, like you, who have overcome similar challenges to those you face. These inspirational women generously share their stories, tried and tested strategies, hints and tips to encourage you to have belief in yourself, your dreams and ambitions.

Designed for busy women like you, I invite you to dip in and out of its pages whenever you feel in need of a dose of inspiration, an uplifting quote or a helpful exercise. Let what you read bring you back to a stronger sense of confidence and self-belief as you move forward, step by step, and confidently overcome those unexpected obstacles. Unpack your shiny new plates; stack them in an orderly pile to serve up something special when required.

1

The Power of Books

As a committed reader from a young age, I understand the magical power of books; their ability to capture the essence of inspirational stories, and form an emotional connection with the reader to help women like you to feel they are not alone.

I originally found the inspiration to publish this book after listening to one of the contributing authors, Natasha Black, recounting passionately her own incredible story of how she transformed herself from a young woman driven by the lure of money and success, to become an inspirational spiritual healer.

Her life experiences were in stark contrast to my own, which until then consisted of an unexceptional career in government agencies and the civil service. Yet, I felt a powerful energetic connection as she spoke, and shared the same desire to break free of the faulty thinking that held me back, much of it formed in childhood.

Several years on from publication of the first edition of this book, I am heartened to receive ongoing feedback about the benefits women have found from reading *Believe You Can Succeed*. Imagine how touching it feels when running into an entrepreneur at a networking meeting who exclaims: "I still have your book by my bedside table", or to receive a message from someone who tells me: "I always read your poems when I feel down, and they make me feel better".

My resolve to update and re-release this anthology was strengthened when, in one week, a series of positive messages arrived in my inbox, letting me know that the book had prompted a lot of mindset change work for one reader, and great enjoyment for the others - one wrote: "I have recommended your wonderful book to my local reading group". Another related how: "I was just in the process of setting up my business, and your book helped me to believe it was possible."

Not only that, but one reader, who commented, "your book started me on the road to believing in myself" subsequently contributed her own story to the third volume in the series – *Believe You Can Live a Life You Love at 50+*. What a powerful testament to believing in the power of your own story!

Journaling

On initial publication, I shared how, after discovering the 'morning pages' process – a technique for writing three full A4 sized pages of free-flowing writing immediately after waking each morning, as advocated in Julia Cameron's book, *"The Artist's Way"*, I began to write poetry.

My signature poem, Believe! became my inspiration to find and share my voice, and again features in the introduction to this volume. I have since found the self-belief to publish *I Am Unique*, a book of my own verse, which secured no.1 status in its category on Amazon!

I had the pleasure of presenting a copy of that book to Julia Cameron herself at a workshop she led in 2017. I highly recommend buying a new journal and using it to write out your thoughts, whether using the morning pages technique or in response to the exercises in this book.

Since first publication, I have developed an inspirational Believe card app, which won a Janey Love's Gold Award, and held my first national event: Your Signature Success Story, at which a number of contributing *Believe You Can Succeed* authors, including Natasha Black, Helen Elizabeth Evans and Nicci Bonfanti shared their passion to help others believe in themselves.

It is these kinds of meaningful experiences that I wish for you in your life and business, and also for your clients.

In the same way that Julia Cameron has updated her iconic book, *The Artists Way*, it feels timely to respond to the warm comments received for *Believe You Can Succeed*, and to give it a new lease of life!

A sense of knowing

Back in 2012, when I first had the grain of an idea to publish an inspirational book of true stories, listening to and following my intuition was fairly new to me.

Nevertheless, whenever it felt right to ask someone to contribute their story to the collection, I committed to do so. I let go of any sense of expectation – my firm belief was that "if they were meant to be in the book, they would be in the book." As such, drawing the stories and contributions of poetry together proved remarkably seamless. The original contributions are a testament to the universal nature and ongoing power of stories - they have stood the test of time.

For this updated version of *Believe You Can Succeed*, my intuition called me to invite 5 additional women to add their inspirational stories.

Jackie Wilson blew me away with her uplifting energy as she related passionately how she had overcome crippling childhood shyness to "put herself out of the equation" when taking forward her incredible mission to help children with their emotional well-being.

Babita Devi is also enhancing the life of children through her amazing app designed to build stronger communities and connection between parents.

Buckso Dhillon-Woolley demonstrates how it is possible to achieve what can seem like a distant dream of success as an actress through determination, and to run a business alongside to help others find their voice.

Jo Roberts bravely recounts her heart-wrenching and very personal experiences around miscarriage and fertility.

Sarah Presley adds inspiration by relating how she faced a diagnosis of M.E. and discovered meditation and reiki.

Keep following the signs

Since writing the Believe! poem, with its opening rallying call to: "Stand up! Stand Up! Be bold, be strong" it has continued to act as a clarion call to me and other women. It spurs me on to develop my vision of inspiring women, particularly the quieter ones who, like me, don't find it easy to find their voice. The words from the poem were instrumental in my initial realisation that I was meant to nurture and grow the nascent *"Believe You Can Succeed"* collection.

After I began to share the idea of the poem and the book in a natural, unforced way other people were inspired to share in my vision. This subsequently led me to produce two further volumes of stories, *Believe You Can Face Your Fears and Confidently Claim the Life You Desire*, and *Believe You Can Live a Life You Love at 50+.*

The seed is planted

Now, let's journey back in time to that mystical moment when the Believe! poem was birthed, easily and effortlessly one crisp March morning.

Visualise, if you will, an unsuspecting middle-aged woman, in a faux grey fur dressing gown, idly browsing the messages on her computer screen. Next, watch with wonder, as a magnetic pull charges from her brain, through her body, to her fingers. Opening a new window on the screen, these fingers begin to fly across the keys, as a poem, addressed to herself, swiftly stakes its claim on the stark whiteness of a blank Word document.

She sits stunned, as a spiritual "wake-up" call stares back at her from the screen. In a matter of minutes, a mystical energy had caught her imagination; sparking her latent creativity and culminating in the creation of her poem:

BELIEVE!

Sue, stand up, stand up! Be bold, be strong!
Your talent, on world stage, truly does belong!
You are a beacon, shining bright,
Birthed to emerge, grow, and shine your inner light!

It is a crime to leave talent, dusty on a rickety, hidden shelf,
Set out your stall; allow true expression
of your amazing inner self.
Surely, you will experience some discomfort as you stretch,
far better than staying a self-defeating, self-pitying little wretch?
Rather, as you experience movement,
create life-changing shifts,
you will, newly emboldened, dare to share your gifts!

Life is truly meant for us to live; by our own example, given
To those, like us, who have sometimes been
Squashed, ignored, or diligently working;
self-effacing, behind a screen
Of uniformity; water poured on burning fire,
Quashed down, made damp squib of all passion and desire.
And, as others bask in your new golden glow,
It helps for them, also to know,
That they have their own miracles to perform,
Whether on a stage, or as more often is the norm,

In their own families and communities,
through their daily life and deeds,
Do great work; sow and nurture the seeds
Of positivity, purposefulness and joy,
With which we all entered this world to buoy
Up ourselves and others,
manifest the birth right of our mothers,
As we mix with friends, many others,
who enter into our life's stratosphere.

All add dark and shade, maybe cause us to shed a tear,
Perhaps of joy or sometimes pain,
so, ultimately, of our own truth, understanding we gain.
Right here and now, we need to show,
Through heartfelt determination,
strength of courage,
We all have the power to foster our own abilities, to grow;
Achieve our birth right to succeed; root out the dreaded weed
That with stranglehold choked down
our well-intentioned schemes,
Left us struggling with dashed hopes, and broken,
once beautiful dreams.

So meaning-full, join us to create,
an interwoven, brilliant picture to which all can relate!
As one voice, stand up and state:

"We are here to live mindfully in this life,
we choose creativity, positive intent over unrewarding strife
and as we choose to change how we ourselves perceive,
in our own dreams, our legacy, our power, we truly believe!"

~ Sue Williams ~

RECOGNISING THAT BUSINESSES HAVE THE POWER TO CHANGE LIVES
~ *Paul Dunn*

"The greater the obstacle, the more glory in overcoming it." — Molière.

In April 2006 a series of events happened that changed the course of my life. Whilst visiting Bangalore, a friend invited me to dinner and introduced me to a man called Pastor Silva.

I recall that first conversation so well. After all, only an Australian could ask "Is that 'Pasta' as in P A S T A or P A S T O R?"

Over a very limited dinner, Pastor Silva recounted how, in 2002 he had taken a trip to set up a church in a small community on an island off the coast of India.

"Everything was going well," he said. "But one Sunday morning just after Christmas Day everything changed."

The reference to a Sunday morning just after Christmas Day should have given me the clue as to what was coming. But it didn't. It's amazing how quickly we forget things.

He continued, "During Sunday school at the church there was this sudden loud noise; the loudest I'd ever heard. I rushed outside and saw a wall of water sweeping towards us. I ran back into the Sunday school trying to keep calm.

9

And I told the 12 children we should play a game in which we would all join hands and run to the high ground."

"We did this. And then with six children either side of me, we stood on the high ground and watched as the church crumpled like a matchbox and was washed away. And then we stood there and saw the children's parents being washed away too."

This was, of course, the devastating tsunami of 2004.

Pastor Silva took the next 18 months to find a place to rehouse the children. "It's been challenging," he said. "And now they need food, insurance, schooling and school books."

I asked him if he'd figured out how much that would cost. "Oh yes," he said, "your friend has been helping me work that out. And it's US$3,500."

"That's per child," I said.

"Oh no, that's for all 12."

If you would have been in my place then, you'd have done precisely what we did – figure out ways to get the funds to them. And we did.

Five weeks later I had an email I'll treasure forever. Pastor Silva had been down to an Internet café, he'd managed to borrow a camera and attach just four photos to the email. Three photographs showed the new home and its environs; the children eating inside, and the side room with the kids and their new school books. But the fourth picture changed everything for me. It was a close-up of the house, and across the top the kids and Pastor Silva had written in large letters "Paul Dunn Home".

In that moment I experienced a sort of epiphany. Until that point, I had thought that business was all about having fun and adding value; those were the only two things I knew. At that moment I realised there was something else. You know how it is, when a sudden insight allows you to see the world in a different way.

And what's really interesting is that the moment you start seeing the world differently, different things start to show up in your life.

So, not surprisingly now in hindsight, just three months later at a workshop in Bali, I met my friend, Masami Sato, again. We'd met briefly before in Brisbane where we both lived at that time. I knew she was a Japanese chef who'd always started businesses with the sole idea of giving back. And I knew she had a tiny business providing gluten-free frozen food to supermarkets and delicatessens in Australia.

The session in Bali was a mentoring programme and I was one of four mentors working at high speed with around 200 entrepreneurs like Masami.

Masami came into the mentoring room with a team she'd assembled. She brought with her the packaging for the food. And there on one side was a large starburst graphic. I still remember what it said, "When you buy this nutritious food, you help us support a soup kitchen in India."

Someone in the room (I like to think it was me) said, "Yes, we've heard of 'Buy 1 GET 1', but this is 'Buy 1 GIVE 1'."

We continued the mentoring on that line. And then I progressed to the next "mentee".

Seven days later I'm back in Brisbane. My phone rings. It's Masami. "How you?" she asks in her lovely Japanese accent. "I very good," I respond (you always speak like others do, don't you!).

"Oh, I cannot sleep seven days," she says.

"Why?"

"Because of Buy 1 GIVE 1. Realise that if I let go of food business [I] can create a platform for all businesses to do Buy 1 GIVE 1. [I] realise can create a world that is full of giving. And that [is] a happier world."

"So how [does] that work?" I ask – I'd totally forgotten about it.

"Simple," says Masami. "You buy TV from TV store …"

"STOP, Masami, STOP! If I buy a TV from a store, that store isn't going to give me another TV – as in buy one, give one."

"You not understand," she says. "You buy TV because you want better vision. So how would it be if when you buy TV, someone who has no vision, someone who cannot see, gets the gift of sight."

The thought of this being a real possibility took my breath away.

And so, Masami continued, "Or you buy a coffee, someone gets the gift of life-saving water. Or you sell your book and a tree gets planted."

I think at that time I exclaimed, "Masami, can I be your mentor for the rest of your life!"

Clearly, here was a concept that could seriously impact our world. The challenge was … how do you make it happen?

That took over two years to figure out. We had to deal with questions of selecting projects. How DO you do that in such a way that you only deal with high-integrity projects, yet projects that are really "close to the action" and not just overloaded with expensive infrastructure? And how do you do it sustainably? And how do you do it so it can scale. And how do you do it so that fully 100% of the giving-back goes to where clients want it to go?

It took a LONG time to develop those answers and to develop the B1G1 platform that makes it all possible. But finally, we got it. And today, B1G1 serves as a platform for businesses to realise what Masami Sato conceptualised back in Bali.

In becoming a B1G1 company, an enterprise allocates a fraction of its revenues towards projects of their choosing. This could be anything from a café owner providing drinking water for every cup of coffee sold, to the accounting firm giving goats to Kenyan families for every new client they gain. B1G1 makes it simple for small- to medium-sized companies to make a meaningful difference to the lives of others, enabling the company to choose projects that resonate with its business and its customers.

We've been able to build B1G1 in a totally new way. We describe it this way – its business giving totally redefined.

You see, in any "rich" country, approximately 70% of the economy is powered by small-to-medium-sized enterprises (SMEs); not big corporations. I believe that the root word in corporate social responsibility, "corporate", turns off the SME person. And yet, internally SMEs know that they want to give back, because it's who we are, it's built into our DNA. So B1G1 solves that AND it gives them much, much more too.

B1G1 is about sweeping away everything you knew about charity and business giving; replacing it with a smarter way of giving that is totally transparent and sustainable.

Today, with B1G1, more than 2,300 businesses from 43 different countries have made over 177 million impacts. Although this may seem immense, to me it is only a tiny part of what could be happening. At B1G1, we believe that in the future more and more businesses in the SME sector will want a simple way of doing good, and B1G1 can provide the platform for this.

I believe deeply in the growing trend of individuals and businesses taking on a social cause.

And it's about doing things for a higher purpose. Richard Branson expressed that well when he urged us to, as he put it, "… explore this next great frontier where the boundaries between work and higher purpose are merging into one, where doing good really is good for business."

And then more recently he added, "I truly believe that businesses that don't address social responsibility and, more importantly, don't put this at the heart of their operations, will suffer over the medium to long term."

The point about "at the heart" is the real key. Of that I'm certain.

Until 2006 I never understood that. Understanding it now has changed my life, and thankfully, the lives of many others as well.

Your beliefs can do the same. Go search for them. Ask yourself relentlessly, "Why do I get up in the morning?" Go deeply until the lump that forms in your throat becomes too big for you to answer the question.

And then live that belief with passion. You'll be living on purpose. You'll be flowing, flourishing and fantastic. And you'll be enjoying and learning from each moment. Go do that now. You'll love it.

Paul Dunn
Chairman of B1G1
More information at www.b1g1.com

I BELIEVE IN MYSELF
Wendy Cotton

I believe in myself,
My roots grow deep,
My branches spread wide and touch the sky.

I believe in myself,
I am transformed in love
My emotions are real and dreams take flight.

THE UNIVERSE HAS YOUR BACK
~ Natasha Black

"Dreams cannot be caught but they can be let in" Natasha Black

I don't know about you but I'm totally driven by my work.

Long ago, my drive was more of a work hard, play hard ethic. Money meant happiness and I wanted lots of both. I was working in property sales in southern Spain seven days a week, earning six figures and I was the top female salesperson pursuing a manager's position and nothing was going to stop me from getting it.

Because that's what I did. I was a self-motivated go-getting doer; life was all about the work and the money and the material possessions at the end of it. Some people would say I was an alpha female – just the thought of it makes me squirm, but it's true!

After a while it became a struggle to keep up the pace and without realising it, I had burned myself out. My boyfriend at the time was pretty keen for me not to work and so I stopped working.

Whilst I revelled in the luxury, there was a part of me that didn't feel comfortable not working. Over time, my boyfriend became even more controlling and abusive in many ways. I ended up hitting rock bottom at the age of 30 and felt like my life was over.

Slowly rebuilding my life, I started to make conscious changes which supported me, but I was still on an unconscious quest for happiness. I had started working again but I was tired of the hard sales environment and longed to get away from it. I became more depleted, more miserable and questioned more and more what I was doing with my life.

I wanted to make a difference in people's lives, in a fulfilling job which made me happy on an inner level rather than on the surface. I'd often write on bits of paper "I want a career I love" and then wrack my brains for what that could be and seemingly get nowhere.

Without realising it, I'd told the Universe many times and in several ways that I was ready to discover my purpose. And with the good old Law of Attraction at work, I was sent a book which would change the course of my life forever. The well-known book "The Secret", by Rhonda Byrne, gave me enough ammunition to go deeper into myself and off I went on an unexpected and amazing journey of self-discovery.

Within six months my life didn't just change; it transformed, and in a radical fashion! I was no longer the person I used to be and I LOVED IT. One of the biggest changes was in my health; for years I had suffered with many illnesses and physical pain. I had headaches every day which sometimes turned into debilitating migraines.

There was always something wrong with me – colds, sinus infections, flu, hay fever, asthma, sickness. My immune system was so weak that I would catch pretty much anything that was going. Then there were the problems with my back, knees, neck, shoulders... I was constantly visiting my chiropractor and getting adjusted but never really being fixed.

But the sickness and physical pain which I had come to believe would never go away seemed to disappear overnight. This was a revelation, especially since I never specifically set out to heal my body. I stopped feeding off drama and filled my life with nourishing people.

My outlook on life was completely different and my thoughts were more positive and supportive. I had a new drive in me and I was "bouncing off the walls", wanting to share what I'd learned with anyone and everyone.

I could hardly believe it, but my inner belief that there was more to life than what I had been experiencing was true. Inherently I knew happiness was attainable and, finally, I had discovered that to have happiness on a deep level, I needed to get to know myself like never before and work through the challenges that lay before me.

Once I knew what I was here to do, my "old" job had to go so that I could start working for myself on my own terms. I had no idea how I was going to do it, but the drive was immeasurable. I knew I had what it would take to make it work.

After all, I had created a very successful six-figure sales career for myself, so why should this be any different?

Within no time I was running regular workshops teaching people how they could change their lives and enjoy more happiness, fulfilment and success. I was speaking at different groups and events. I had a steady rate of one-on-one clients, mainly through referrals, and I was being interviewed on radio shows, Internet TV and had started my own Internet radio show interviewing some really great names. I'd even started my own business networking group and a Law of Attraction group, which were both a great success.

My eyes were firmly fixed on the goal and I went hell for leather to get my name and work out there to the masses. And I did well, very well. Next, I decided it was time to ramp it up big time and went into over-drive. My goal was to get my message out to as many people as possible in the shortest time possible. I did what I did best and used every ounce of my drive and determination to get me there.

Except this time it didn't work.

The old way of doing things had stopped working.

This goal-getting strategy which I'd created for myself no longer got me the goal. I have to say I was quite perplexed. The more I chased my dream, the more it eluded me. I started to make really crap decisions which ended up in mistakes and costly ones at that. I thought I was listening to my intuition, but for some reason the more stuff I tried the less it seemed to work.

I'd been on such an incredible journey; my life had transformed and I was helping people all over the world to transform their lives too. So why on earth was it so difficult to take my work and my business to the next level? I knew what I wanted and I wasn't scared of hard work. I'd read so many books, had done tons of courses, and I had spent thousands to be on a 12-month mastermind programme in America. I seemed to be pushing all the right buttons but nothing would get me any further than where I was!

The more I pursued my dream, the more desperate I became to achieve it, which left me feeling an all too familiar unhappiness. In just a couple of short months of feeling this way, my business came to a halt. I was getting married, fell pregnant the month before and moved country. This was exactly what I needed, even though it didn't feel like it at the time.

During and after my pregnancy I took on a small number of clients and felt pretty desperate to get back into work the way I had been used to. I struggled with my identity as a mum for quite a few months – I'd gone from being a well-known transformational coach and mentor in Brussels, Belgium, to practically being wiped off the map in a work capacity.

In my head, I was constantly thinking about how I was going to get my business going again and I couldn't wait to get childcare in place.

Looking back now, I can hardly believe this was how I was behaving! It was like I was running out of time and had to do this as soon as possible. By the time my daughter was six months old I was working a couple of days a week and felt happy I could now get back into it.

I wanted to continue where I left off and decided to do an event for purpose-driven female entrepreneurs called "Believe – in your Dreams, Legacy and Power". I was really excited to be doing what I knew I was capable of, and set all the wheels in motion. Everything was falling into place and I felt like I kept being guided to the next step.

That is until I started to feel heavy in my head and body and I literally had to stop. I know enough about how the body works, in particular my body, and decided to take a break from the event. I thought I was probably doing too much, especially as I was doing this every day whilst my daughter was taking her naps; during the evenings and on childcare days. In fact, every waking moment was taken up by the event and clearly, I needed a break.

But then, I just couldn't get back into it with the same drive I had had before. It seemed like I'd gone from one extreme to another; from excited to overwhelm and from being in the flow to being filled with anxiety.

It was taking its toll on me and my family and I knew something had to change.

After some help from one of my closest friends, I discovered that I was stuck in my old ways of working, and they no longer suited me. This drive had me chasing my goal as if time was running out; believing that I wanted to work flat out, full time. This was no longer true for me. Yes, I wanted to get my work out to more people, but not like this!

So, I made a really big, tough decision to honour my new wisdom and pulled the plug on what I'd created! The lightness and relief I felt from making that decision was so refreshing that I knew I'd made the right one. From there I was able to gain the insight that this event was still being called to go ahead but on a much smaller scale.

After much deliberation, I invited a group of eight women to attend the Believe Retreat; three days focussing on their growth and transformation as individuals rather than being part of a much larger audience. It was a great success and I was more than delighted with the outcome.

Looking at the event as I'd initially created it, I realised I'd been chasing my dream to the point of exhaustion and this wasn't how I was supposed to behave. From that point on, I decided to take some time out to regroup and focus on me. I knew it was time to let my dream come to me and that nothing I wanted was outside of me. This wasn't a race – I had nowhere to be other than right here, right now. The Universe had my back and it was time to stop taking erratic action and replace it with action with patience. And sometimes this meant doing nothing.

And very quickly everything shifted.

I now take action with patience. There really is no need to chase a goal I've set outside of myself. I know that my dream will be fulfilled and way beyond anything I can believe, perceive or conceive. The Universe has my back and my job is to do the inner work.

And I bring this message to you too, my friends who are on this path with me. Erase erratic action and embrace action with patience, which sometimes includes doing nothing. Your dream will come to you if you let it in!

EXERCISES:

1. Each morning, take between 5-15 minutes before you start your day to breathe in the Universe and its wisdom. Sit in a quiet place, bring your attention to your body, and then let it go. Bring your attention to your heart then let it go. Bring your attention to your mind, and then let it go. Bring your attention to your dream and ask your soul/ higher self to guide you to letting your dream in. The more you do this, the more guidance you will receive and not necessarily just during this quiet time.

2. Remember that time is an illusion of the ego and can trap you into thinking that you must move quickly to achieve instant results. Be consciously aware when you are taking erratic action which is leading you nowhere and immediately bring yourself back to the present, dropping anything which isn't supporting you. Use your new mantra many times a day "There is nowhere I need to be, other than right here, right now. The Universe has my back and wants me to take action with patience. I'm letting in my dreams and allowing them to unfold in God's time, not mine."

3. Go on a Rampage of Self-Acknowledgement. Every evening, write a minimum of five things in your journal that you acknowledge and appreciate in yourself for that day. It doesn't matter what they are and they don't have to be big things. Watch how your self-belief grows along with your confidence, when you take the time to recognise yourself.

Natasha Black has a huge desire for personal growth. She says – I know that for me to keep evolving into the very best version of me I can be and to live my best life, I have only one choice and that is to grow personally. I also know that if I want to go beyond what I think is possible, I need the help of the Universe to make it happen. I share what I learn from my own journey in my coaching programs, healing practice, workshops, retreats, writing and speaking.

You can find me at: www.natashablack.net

BELIEVE IN LOVE
Elizabeth Beetham

I am alone

Yet my heart

Sets flight

Imagining a different life

When my belief

Was safe and sure

Within the arms of

He who lived

Now he is gone

I wait in vain

For his clear voice

To call my name

I am alone

Yet filled with love.

I BELIEVE IN LOVE
~ *Elizabeth Beetham*

"I believe in mankind's absolute ability to love." Elizabeth Beetham

Today I will begin. My desire is to inspire. A rather large ambition but I am going to do my best. To change mediocrity in myself and others to a positive belief that anything is possible when we have faith and trust in ourselves. We often need lots of help with this, so first I put my faith and trust in God – you may not have that belief but many do believe in that higher power or spirit who in my opinion so surely guides our lives.

To relish and find joy in life is my quest for you all. Just being sure and confident that when we express love to ourselves and others, we are fulfilling our true purpose can bring joy so easily to our lives. This is not to say that it is always easy to feel joy or love. Life can be very challenging at times; every one of us experiences sadness and pain at some time during our life's journey.

There will always be times when we falter and struggle, not knowing exactly what to do and where we should go. I am sure most of us have experienced the urge to run away. I certainly have. When my husband died suddenly of a heart attack, I did physically run away and hid from the world for almost a year. I went and lived in a different place; but we cannot truly run away because "even in paradise we take ourselves!"

28

Let me explain this little saying – it means that we cannot run away from who we truly are. We can never really run away from ourselves or indeed the circumstances we find ourselves in. It is only when we start to understand ourselves, who we are and our motives behind our patterns of behaviour that we can find peace and happiness. To really love, you must first learn to love yourself. Not of course in a selfish way, but in an accepting way. No one is perfect after all, and once we realise this, not only does it help to forgive other people's imperfections but more importantly our own.

Losing anyone you love is devastating and something we are so ill-equipped to deal with. As someone said when my husband died, we are not good at facing the inevitability of death.

I had no idea that John was going to die. He did have high blood pressure and had seen a heart consultant, but he seemed fine. With hindsight, I realise now how ill he was, but he didn't want me to know; his fitness was part of his pride, part of who he wanted to be. He even went climbing in the Brecon Beacons just prior to Christmas. John was never happier than when he was climbing a mountain. Christmas was really lovely that year. In fact, he said it was one of our best. Little did we know it was the last we would spend together.

New Year: we were in Devon with all my siblings and we danced the New Year in, laughing and feeling excited about what 2010 would bring! On 2 January we were travelling to stay with friends and I was driving. John seemed a bit on edge, impatient as we were diverted. As I was trying to park the car in Totnes, he got out to try and find a parking space. Another car moved out a little behind, and while I was concentrating on parking, John had a massive heart attack. He stopped breathing a few times. On 6 January he died in hospital in Devon and a part of me died too.

I felt destroyed, desolate. The happy carefree person I was, who felt safe in the surety of unconditional love, died that day. John adored me and spoilt me. He was a good man, a gentleman. I was so fortunate to find him and spend nearly twenty years with him. We had a great life together; not that he didn't drive me mad at times! I am sure he found me difficult at times too. I miss him so much that I am crying now writing this, but I want you to recognise that the important thing is to appreciate the ones we love, and tell them how much we love them while they are still here.

When someone dies, we have to learn how to live a new life without them and transport that love we experienced while they were alive into our new life. We must all leave this earth – it is our only certainty. How we decide to live is our choice, but first we need to grieve.

My experience of grieving has been truly awful; a heart-wrenching process, but necessary. It is often something you can't control. I have stood in Marks & Spencer crying at the checkout because I am buying flowers – John always bought me flowers. There are some days when you don't want to get out of bed – there seems no point. Regret floods over you, and you ask why, you analyse everything that happened and try to make sense of it.

And there are days when you feel so angry you want to shout and fight everyone and everything. Days when you cry so much you feel there are no more tears to shed; but there always are.

It may be a piece of music, or a photograph, or a smell that sets you off again. I won a raffle on Valentine's Day and stood and cried in the department store because I felt John had sent me a present that day. Once, when I went running, tears flowed as I stopped to cross the road; I saw a two pence coin on the ground. John used to call me "tuppence" – another message that he is still near me. It is amazing how often I have found two pence coins since he died. Life is full of mystery that we do not and probably should not understand.

It is almost three years now. Some days I feel the worst is over. We do adapt and we do learn to go on. What you come to realise is that you can never overcome your loss. As time goes by you simply learn to live with it. If you are recently bereaved then my advice is to keep busy and be open to help from your family and friends. My running away now feels wrong. I distanced myself from the people who love me because I did not know how to be honest about my grief. I did not want them to see my grief.

The first six months I spent a lot of time alone trying to come to terms with my loss. The one thing I did that really helped was yoga. I had an excellent yoga teacher who came to the flat I was living in. We worked hard but also talked and I learned not to fight the sadness. I learned to accept it. There is an old saying – what we resist persists, and I believe that to be true.

Feeling sad day in, day out was such an alien feeling, but with the help of my yoga teacher I learnt acceptance and also gratitude for the things I still have in my life. What also helped was focussing on the good times we shared and talking about John. He will always be a precious part of my life. Although he is not here, I feel his presence and still feel his love. The life I lead now is different but I can still say I love my life, and I am grateful for my life.

Perhaps we find the secret to a joyful life when we relax and let life flow because in truth, we have no control of life at all. When we let go and let life flow, an easier path can be found and experienced. Even when the going gets tough a deep certainty of purpose can prevail and sustain us.

The never-ending question of the meaning of life can never be answered. We are life. Life is being experienced through and within us. Life is our gift to us and as such it is precious beyond measure. What we do with this gift is entirely our own choice.

Life is about choice. Every day when we open our eyes, we make a choice. Will I smile and count my blessings today and be happy with what I have? Or will I be miserable and dwell on all the things I don't have in my life? My experience has taught me the importance of being grateful for life and all its gifts. On rare occasions I have touched that evasive feeling of true contentment and it has always been in those moments of feeling true gratitude for this wonderful world.

When we have faith and believe in our future, then that future will bring us all we desire, because we choose the life we want. Every day we make that choice. I urge you to choose and believe in joy and happiness.

Make a list of all the things you are grateful for and read that list every day. You will soon discover the pleasure your life already holds for you. It does not have to be anything complicated; just a short list of the things that bring you happiness. I have found this exercise can truly change how you feel about your life.

The fundamental experience of life teaches us that we are many things and each separate aspect of our character is purely the reflection of the moment and the choices we have made.

Right now, I wish to be a teacher, I want to help and improve your life's journey. I want to help you believe in yourself. Because my friend, life is passing in a flash, so we need to seize the day. I had to believe in myself or I would not have carried on. I had to believe that my being here in the world was worthwhile. I had to believe I could make a positive difference. This belief, fostered by self-analysis and self-development books and courses I have attended over the years has helped me enormously. Anthony Robbins' "Unleash the Power Within" was life-changing. After that course I changed my work and did a degree in nutrition.

Search and find out what you want out of life. What is your passion? You really have to learn to understand yourself to really give of yourself. I still have lots to learn but working with people and helping them is the most important part of my life now.

What I have come to understand and believe is that we all have a tremendous capacity to find joy in the everyday experience of just living. One of the keys is not to compete, so give up comparing your life with someone else's. It's silly; we all get it so wrong at times. Life is not a competition and complaining about your lot will certainly not bring you happiness, only misery. I desire you to choose joy, choose happiness. I want you to believe that joy is a natural part of your life from now and forever.

Life is wonderful. Just sit for a moment and think about all the things you have done so far in your life. All those people whose lives you have touched. It really is miraculous. Holidays, homes, hotels, hospitals, horrendous relatives – all the stuff that has made up your life so far. Wow, isn't it amazing you have survived?

Relax. Yes, despite Facebook, Twitter, iPhones, television, particularly all the bad news, the Internet and the whole catastrophe of the modern world, at times we all need to simply step back and just chill! Be with who you really are right now in this moment. There are actually no winners in life and indeed no losers; only "faulty thinking" makes us believe there are.

The past does not equal the future unless you live there. You can change your life anytime you are ready. Small changes make a big difference and it's really all about attitude. It is all about belief in yourself and that magical ability to identify what you really want. You can do this – it just takes a little courage and a lot of love.

Look at all the areas of your life: your work, your health and your relationships. Do you love your job, and if not why not? What can you do to change it? Do you need a new career path and what steps do you need to take to change how you feel? Have you held on to some old worn-out belief about yourself that is not true today?

Start to be kind to yourself – be your own best friend. Have you festered some disagreement with a family member for so long that you cannot remember what actually happened? Forgive and forget the past, send love and heal that hurt before it is too late.

To understand where we are, we have to answer some difficult questions. As I said, we have to be brave to make change happen in our lives. We have to believe in our ability to live a joyful and happy life. Happiness is there for us all, so believe in yourself and give love.

EXERCISES:

1. It is important to ask for what you want in life. As Jesus said "Ask and it will be given." I use affirmations and encourage my clients to use affirmations, to harness the power to change things in their lives. An affirmation is a statement of the truth of something. You can use them to bring that truth into your life right now. Write your statements of truth in a journal or diary. As you write them down say them out loud. Read and write them repeatedly until you feel that you have received that truth.

2. I work with many women to help them to gain control of their mind, body and often their weight, which is a major issue in the Western world, where we are blessed with plenty. The first affirmation I give them is "I am a slim person!" Yes, they often laugh, especially if they are obese, but many soon begin to realise the power of that affirmation!

As we write down our affirmations, they become part of our subconscious and part of our life. They are a very powerful tool for bringing change into your life. There are many mysteries which we do not understand. I believe affirmations are part of the mystery of life. They are truly an amazing way of transforming your life. Start today and find the difference they can make for you.

The following are three affirmations I use to help me with my self-belief, to help me live the best life I can. You can use these or make up your own. Affirmations must be statements, things you want right now. Write them as if you are already experiencing them and have received the gifts already. They are strong statements of intent.

1. I forgive myself and my enemies and now I am free. With God on my side, who can be against me?

2. I awake and feel joy and gratitude for my life.

3. I breathe peace and love into my heart.

Elizabeth Beetham is a nutritionist, health journalist, broadcaster, public speaker and well-being expert. Colleagues and clients describe her as inspirational and innovative as well as resourceful and enthusiastic.

Contact Elizabeth at www.powerforhealth.com

BELIEVE IN LIFE
Elizabeth Beetham

Believe, you have a choice
Choose life
Joy and pain
Beauty and ugliness
Must exist
Without both we are blind

To taste sweetness
Life must first sour the tongue
The answer is
Accept, for everything passes.

THE GIFT
~ *Floyd Carlson*

"*We are what we repeatedly do. Excellence, then, is not an act, but a habit.*" Aristotle

In everyone's life there are one or many opportunities, challenges or situations that become a catalyst to change a person's life. In Elise Ballard's book "Epiphany", she provides a vehicle for many people to tell their stories about that key incident that changed their life. She defines an epiphany as "a moment of great or sudden revelation; an intuitive grasp of reality through something unusually simple and striking; an illuminating discovery, realization, or disclosure".

When we look at our own lives and focus on what moments made a difference, we will find our own epiphany. My opportunity occurred in the war in Iraq during Operation Desert Storm. It became my life-changing event that has taken me on an amazing journey and transformation.

Iraq – day 3 of the ground offensive of Operation Desert Storm (Tuesday 26 February 1991). I was a first lieutenant with Bravo Company 4/7 Infantry and I was the unit's Executive Officer. Since the ground offensive had begun, we were constantly on the move and in frequent engagement with Iraqi forces. On this particular day we were fighting against the Metadine Republican Guard and this day would have a profound impact on my life and the future direction I would follow.

The sky was black from the burning oil well fires and throughout the day and night everything was a blur. My company was deployed on line and firing at targets to our

39

front and all around us. I remember the ground being littered with destroyed equipment and ammunition. The sounds of explosions and the firing of weapons were happening all around me.

I could see my company commander's vehicle off to my left as my vehicle started up an incline, when Castro my driver yelled out "Sniper ahead!" The sniper had my commander in his line of fire when I first saw him. I instantly began to push down on my firing trigger to take him out. At this moment he turned and we both were staring directly at each other.

It was as if the world stood still. A tunnel encapsulated us both and everything was moving in slow motion. It felt as though I was watching an old western gun fight scene, except I was in it and this was a matter of life and death. Without hesitation there was no play left in my trigger and I was squeezing the last bit of pressure needed to complete the task. With our eyes locked on each other, he did something I did not expect. He threw his weapon to the ground, went on his knees and began to pray out loud to Allah. My finger released the grip I had on my trigger. Neither of us was to die that day.

Castro covered me and kept his weapon aimed on this man, who was now lying on the ground, as I jumped out of our vehicle and went to get the other four Iraqi soldiers out of their fighting position. Soon the five men were lying on the ground as I started to check each one for weapons. When I was checking one of the men, I made a fatal mistake.

As a soldier we are trained to search prisoners of war by lying on the ground next to them and reaching over and searching them from behind. The reason is that if they are booby-trapped with an explosive device, we can roll them on top of it and hopefully not kill ourselves in the process.

As I was checking the man with whom just a few minutes ago I was in a mortal stare down, I felt something next to his chest that did not feel right. Rather than rolling him on top of it, I pulled it out and saw a black cylinder tube with wires coming out of the top and heard a distinct sound I knew very well, a thud. This was the sound of a round or charge going down a tube to a firing pin. My body completely shut down and I said to myself "I'm dead."

I have heard stories that when you know you are about to die your life flashes before your eyes. This is completely true. As I believed I was dead from the critical mistake I had just made, I saw my life in an instant flash before my eyes. I saw images of all the important people in my life from my grandparents, parents, great friends I had, my partner Ellen, and an image of a small blond-haired boy aged about four years old.

At that time Ellen was pregnant and we did not know the sex of our first child. That image I saw would be Eric, our first-born son, and he would look exactly as I had pictured him that day in a flash of my life.

All the images I saw were of people who were at their happiest moment. There were no pictures of possessions or things I had accomplished. Just the key people who had shared my life and one who would be in my life.

I did not fully realise that I had just been given a gift that would transform my life forever. No, I was not dead. The device I had pulled out of his jacket was a homemade radio and the sound I heard was a battery sliding down the tube. This was what we called in the Army a "shorts-changing moment".

It was only many years later that I fully appreciated the gift I had been given that day. Just recalling this, one of many situations that occurred during my deployment for Desert Storm, was very painful. When I told the stories or thought about what had occurred, I would fully relive the events as if they were happening back in Iraq. All the emotions I had felt there were being experienced again in my body. My heart would start to beat faster, my palms would be wet with sweat and my skin colour would go pale. Needless to say, I would bury the memories and pain associated with them.

This was the status quo until I met an amazing coach who would introduce me to two techniques: Emotional Freedom Technique (EFT), which was founded by Gary Craig (www.eftuniverse.com/), and Matrix Reimprinting from Karl Dawson (www.matrixreimprinting.com/). By using these two techniques with me, Natasha Black helped me to have the major breakthrough of actually realising I was still reliving post-traumatic stress from being in combat, and the emotional toll I was carrying because of it.

Awareness is always the first step to unlocking your real potential for a new result. She helped me to find the gift I was given that day in Iraq and see the wisdom it was meant to give me.

The coaching sessions I had with Natasha helped me to release the negative energy and emotions tied to events throughout my life. Each situation where the emotions were released allowed me to learn new things about those

42

events. This included what beliefs and perceptions I had formed around those episodes. The really interesting thing is that as you start the work on yourself, your subconscious begins showing you more and more pictures of moments in your life from which to gain relief and emotional freedom.

After we covered this particular life story from Desert Storm in one of the sessions, I felt as though I had just run a marathon and a huge weight had been lifted from my shoulders. This feeling of relief was invigorating. Now, for the first time, I was able to see the gift and wisdom I had been given.

What was my epiphany? Seeing my life flash before my eyes was all about the great people in my life, not the titles, cars, things, etc. The wisdom I gained was to start with the end of your life in mind and to be the best person I could be by helping others. The questions I began to ask myself and keep a journal on were: what is the legacy I want to leave? What would I like my obituary to say about how I showed up in life? What are the important things I want to achieve?

This was a powerful experience to clearly ground me in what I wanted to become, and in how I wanted to act and be every day. This launched me on my journey to put people first, live life to the fullest, follow my soul's intent and have fun learning new and wonderful things.

I now had a new level of motivation. I wanted to make a positive difference in this world, to be an incredible person and to unlock my full potential. My thoughts turned to where do I start? Looking at one of my strengths, something that had helped me in the past, I used my passion for learning to get me started. This led me on my quest to learn as much as I could and to adopt the items that best fit me into my daily and weekly routines.

I read many books, listened to numerous audio programmes and attended seminars on EFT, Matrix Reimprinting, Neuro-linguistic programming (NLP) and the "Unleash the Power Within" event with Tony Robbins in Rome. All of these were amazing experiences and the biggest value was the sensational people I met who were on their own journeys.

What I have found is that when people who have the same focus get together and share their stories, the energy of both people grows and expands. This is such a sensational feeling! Below are the key insights that I have gained which work for me and that are helping me to achieve my goal of making a difference. I encourage each and every one of you to try out the ones that feel right for you and build your own success routines. This is how you will put all of the things together that you have learned in the "Believe!" book, and achieve your own amazing success.

"Be yourself; everyone else is already taken." Oscar Wilde The first insight I want to share is all about how to be you. To help in this area, you need to do the daily inner work on yourself. It is essential for each of us to focus on our inner self to make the changes we want to have in our life. If you want the world to change, you need to change the words you use and the thoughts you have first.

Why is this so critical to master? In her recording on "Heal Negative Charges", 31 October 2010, Ann Taylor (www.innerhealing.com), highlights that the average person has 60,000 thoughts a day and 77% of them are negative. That is a whopping 46,200 non-productive thoughts a person has each day. The kicker is 95% of the thoughts are the same thoughts they had the day before. These negative thoughts and emotions are destructive.

In her book, "You Can Heal Your Life", Louise L. Hay states, "If we are willing to do the mental work, almost anything can be healed." The message this wonderful book provided is that we are each responsible for our own reality and "dis-ease". Her belief is we are making ourselves ill when we have thoughts of self-hatred. The lesson I learned was this is an area I must focus on daily. What do I do?

Every morning I do a scripted EFT routine, followed by listening to Ann Taylor's programme, mentioned above, on "Heal Negative Charges". As I stretch and prepare for my morning run or bike ride, I listen to inspirational audio books on my iPod. Motivational speaker Robin Sharma's belief that the books you read and the people you hang out with, are who you will be in five years, is great encouragement for listening to and reading material that will empower you to achieve your dreams.

During my running or biking exercising (which gives me sensational energy) I do my mental work. I start with my mental review of my code of conduct, which covers the areas that are most important to me in my life. I then mentally review what I am grateful for and my five power questions.

These include a combination of: Who do I love, who loves me and how does that make me feel? What am I committed to? What is wonderful in my life? What am I excited about in my life? What am I really happy about in my life? What will I do today that makes a difference? I then finish with my affirmations. This represents the first 60-90 minutes of my day and sets me up for having a stress-free start, being energized and excited about what I'm going to achieve that day.

Every evening I will spend my last hour of the day disconnecting and preparing. I stay away from email, TV, news, etc. during this hour. I find that if I don't, I end up thinking about these things and it impacts the quality of my sleep.

During this time, I will write in my journal about how my day went, what I was grateful for and acknowledge myself for the items I was really proud of. The secret here is that what you capture in your journal is what you get more of in your life. I will do some more reading and spend at least 15 minutes meditating. I find guided Kundalini yoga meditation from the audio book, "Meditation as Medicine: Activate the Power of Your Natural Healing Force" by Dharma Singh Khalsa, works very well.

In addition, a must-read I recommend to help you with the inner work is "The Big Leap: Conquer Your Hidden Fear and Take Life to the Next Level", by Gay Hendricks. This book helps to identify the "Upper Limit Problem", which is the negative emotional reaction that occurs when anything positive enters people's lives. This limit impacts happiness, prevents us from achieving our goals and is a huge life roadblock.

To make our dreams come true we must each take action and continue to repeatedly follow through until we master the new skill. The second insight is that will power is a muscle that each of us can work on and make stronger. In his book, "The Power of Habit: Why We Do What We Do in Life and Business", Charles Duhigg demonstrates using scientific discoveries why habits exist and how they can be changed. The big idea is that your habits are not your destiny.

My friends will say that my time in the military gave me the discipline to easily do my daily success routines and that it is harder for them because they were not in the services. This is not true and I normally reply that this is just an excuse or limiting belief holding them back. It comes down to just taking action.

A formula I learned from Tony Robbins' time management series, which works well for me, is called OPM. The "O" stands for the outcome you want to achieve. The "P" is for the purpose of why you want that outcome. And the "M" is for the massive action plan you are going to do to achieve your outcome. The two added components that help drive this to be such a success is to measure if you are achieving what you wanted and, if not, to change it.

Every Sunday I will sit down for an hour and plan out my week. Robin Sharma's audio programme and workbook on "Master Your Time, Master Your Life", provides a great process to plan your week and I use his framework. First, I review the plan from the week before and look for the lessons I learned. Reflection is important to gain the wisdom of what works well and doesn't work for me.

I then review my planning book I made in this order: my vision board (all those pictures and words of what I want to achieve in my life); my 14 intentions of what I want to achieve before I die; my living my dream commitment (my purpose statement, code of conduct, my big dream statement, my why I want it and my commitments); my life plan (4 personal & 4 professional categories); long-term goal chart (3 bullets for personal & professional goals for 1, 3, 5 & 10 years); and finally my 90-day goals for my personal & professional life.

This makes me very focused on what I need to do to achieve these goals and what is most important to me. Now I plan out my week and the goals I want to achieve. For each goal I use the OPM structure to ensure I am extremely clear on what I want as my outcome, why I want it and what actions I will take to achieve it.

The next step is very important. I schedule my activities in my calendar to support my weekly plan. The best way to get something completed is to schedule it. What you schedule gets done. I then do a daily brief review of my weekly plan to keep my focus and energy flowing to those most important life goals.

Why do I work and focus on these success strategies daily? The gift that I was given and the journey this has sent me on continues to be rewarding for me every day. My investment, doing the inner work, being disciplined and following through has given me incredible confidence and courage. I am happier; I'm following my life purpose and my dream daily. This has been the biggest transformation in my life and the results have been great.

I recently received a big promotion in my job, I have a stronger relationship with my loved ones and every day I have a great outlook on life. I owe so much of my success, happiness and growth to Natasha Black, who helped me to unlock my full potential with her coaching. She helped me to realise that the epiphany on the battle field in Iraq on that particular day sent me on my path to tell my story and change my life. This was a true game changer. I encourage each and every one of you to look inside yourself to find your key moment of transformation and tell your great personal story. This will be your catalyst to achieve and live the amazing life you and your soul are meant to live. Be the incredible person you are destined to be and believe in your dream!

EXERCISES:

The three exercises below are to reinforce the big ideas from my journey I have shared with you.

1. Find your epiphany and story
What is that moment in your life that sparked your transformation?

Just as reading a book is a conversation you have with the author, keeping a journal is the same as having a conversation with yourself. The purpose of this exercise is to begin your habit of taking time daily to think about your story, your successes and all the other great things that you want to manifest in your life. What you focus on is where your energy flows. Your action: if you do not already have a journal, go out and get one.

Use your journal as your transformation agent to help you make the changes you want in life. Spend 10 minutes a day to go deep within and answer these questions:

What is my epiphany?

What wisdom can I gain from this game-changing moment?

What are my gifts?

What legacy do I want to leave?

What three actions can I take today that will bring me closer to the legacy I want to leave?

Being a victim versus adopting a responsible mind-set
Begin the inner work to become the best version of you. How you view the world and show up every day is essential to your transformation and success. Your language and mind-set play such an important role in your personal success. Are you playing the role of a victim or are you acting as if you are responsible for your actions and what happens to you?

A victim frame of mind means that you give up your control and feel that the things happening to you are beyond your own influence. Whereas adopting a responsible framework means you believe you are an active player in every situation based on your actions.

This exercise is adopted from a session I attended with the Trium Group. The purpose of this exercise is to understand how you feel when you are acting victimised as compared to when you take control and are being responsible for what happens to you.

First pick one of your stories where you feel you were a victim and tell this story for five to ten minutes to a friend, family member, partner, peer, etc. Tell the story with all the emotion of how you felt this other person wronged you. After you have completed your tale, ask the person you just shared this with, on a scale of one to ten (one low, ten high), how convincing were you with how you were victimised.

In your journal or on a piece of paper, write about how you feel. This can be just adjectives, bullets or a paragraph. The essential part is capturing the feelings and the state you are in now.

It is now time to tell the exact same story for five to ten minutes to a friend, family member, partner, peer, etc; except this time, you tell the story where you are fully responsible for the outcome and what happened during this exchange.

Yes, this sounds difficult and you are probably thinking "How could I have been responsible for what they did to me?"

Stick with it and tell the story from this new perspective. Same as last time, once you have finished, ask the person you just shared this with, on a scale of one to ten (one low, ten high), how convincing you were with how you took responsibility for what had occurred.

Next to the items you captured after you told the story as a victim, write about how you now feel after taking responsibility.

Compare the two, reflect and write in your journal on: what wisdom have you just gained from this exercise? How do you feel when you act as if you are responsible versus playing the victim? Which one will help you to unlock your full potential? What will you change when moving forward? Now commit to what you have just decided to do when moving forward.

2. Take action with the 90/28 rule
The best way to start building your will power muscle is to take action and follow through.

The moment you have a new idea, goal or direction, take some sort of action towards its achievement within 90 seconds. This could be ordering a new book, making an appointment with a coach, brainstorming an action plan, or anything else that will start you on the path to making it happen.

The second part of the rule is to do it for 28 straight days to make your new goal and commitment a habit. It is critical to stick with this habit to make it part of your success routine.

The purpose of this exercise is to make a commitment, take some sort of action within 90 seconds and do it 28 straight days to make it an integral part of what you do.

3. From what you have read in this "Believe!" book, keep a journal on what three commitments you promise yourself to achieve in the next six months. By each of these promises, list the outcome, purpose and action steps you will take to make these happen. Within 90 seconds pick one and do it.

Now make your dreams come true by doing the things you want to be part of your daily success routine for the next 28 days.

Have fun and enjoy your journey and the gift your epiphany has given you!

Floyd Carlson is a Corporate Executive and certified coach with over 30 years of experience leading teams, mentoring and coaching people. You can connect with him on LinkedIn. http://www.linkedin.com/

FOR HER
Donna Smith

Life didn't teach her to dream or believe
so, I did it for her
Life brought her fear and shame and pain
so, I believed for her again
Life tore out her heart and took it away
so, I believed harder and stronger
for her to believe
For her to believe that life could be
loving and fair and free
but she couldn't yet see
So, I believed again

I kept believing when it hurt me,
when it took my strength
but I had been lucky, my life had showed me
love and faith and commitment
so, I knew how to keep believing
and then believe some more
So, I did it for her again
I did it out of the sheer unfairness that
life can be so cruel to some
whilst lavishing others
with everything a soul would desire
I did it to balance some sort of karmic debt
that I had been so fortunate
and she had not
Then I believed some more

Then I noticed that in her eyes
there was a tiny spark of belief,
maybe it would grow
maybe it would falter
in the years of pain
now was the greatest test of all for me
To believe
To let go

To let go and let her
believe for herself
that life could be kind
I believe I can do it,
I have to
because life itself depends on it.

Belief is personal,
it is not a given
it is to be taught, awakened,
learned, earned
but when it is achieved it
allows you to live life to its fullest
to breathe, to fly, to be free
Life wants that for her too
I believe.

TIME TO BLOSSOM
~ *Dr Michelle Clarke*

"And the day came when the risk to remain tight in a bud was more painful than the risk it took to blossom." Anaïs Nin

"Discovering your Zone of Genius is your life's Big Leap. Everything up until now has been about hops, not leaps. Hopping, though it seems safe, is actually hazardous to your health. If you confine yourself to hops, you run the risk of rusting from the inside out." Gay Hendricks

A few years ago, I attended my very first conference for coaches. I wasn't a coach at the time – I was an academic, a soil scientist. I'd spent 15 years studying and building up a career that saw me spending my days discussing environmental and soil protection policies with government officials, doing fieldwork (digging holes and examining soil) and working in labs wearing a white coat and goggles.

At times it was exciting. At times I felt like I was making a difference and serving the planet. And at times I felt like I was merely putting in the hours in order to get through the week. I had this little voice that used to whisper to me that there was something else out there, that used to let me know I wasn't using all of my strengths, that reminded me (infrequently at first, and then almost daily) that there was more to me and that I wasn't doing myself or anyone else any favours by not exploring further.

But I guess I need to rewind a bit further. I didn't really become aware of personal development until my early thirties. I spent my twenties studying to get three degrees, and finally got my PhD aged 28. I moved into an academic research post and continued to research and work on different projects. I was happy and engaged with my work, and living very much in my head – reading and writing academic papers, analysing data, producing reports. I was constantly surrounded by piles of paper and books from the library.

It was during this time that the voice started. It was pretty quiet at first and I ignored it easily – I felt it was a natural thing to feel after studying for so long – surely, I was just adjusting to "work" and finding my place within the academic community? I found when I was busy working with a team of people the voice was quieter, and when I worked alone it got louder. When I had flexibility in how I created my day it would leave me in peace, and when I was stuck behind a computer or in the lab it would start to shout!

Around that time, I was sent on some management training courses – most of these were deathly dull, but one introduced me to Neuro-linguistic programming (NLP... a posh way of saying the "science of what makes people tick"). After that day's course I felt everything start to change!

I wanted to know more about NLP, so I followed up with a Business Practitioner course and absorbed everything I could about the subject like a sponge. The simple acceptance that I was responsible for my life, that I had choices, and that I could take action to change things that weren't the way I wanted them to be, was incredibly powerful.

I started integrating what I was learning into my own life – I got promoted and doubled my salary within 18 months (highly unusual within the academic career ladder!). I proposed to my partner (after waiting for nine years for him to propose to me ☺), found better relationships with those closest to me, and better understood relationships that weren't working and my role in helping them to improve. I also started sharing what I was learning with others – friends and colleagues over a coffee – and saw the difference it was having in their lives too.

The next couple of years were wonderful – my own growth was increasing, I was able to support others within the university with their development; the projects I was working on were exciting, and my confidence within my role increased dramatically. I got married, renovated a gorgeous house, and became a mum. Life was good.

I went on maternity leave feeling like I'd turned things around and silenced the voice inside. I had nine blissful months with my little boy – learning to be a mum and cherishing our time together.

When the time came to go back to work, I realised very quickly that the voice hadn't gone anywhere. What I had started to call "the still small voice within" was louder now than it had ever been! I realised that if I was choosing to work instead of being with my son, then the work I was doing had to fulfil me in a way I'd never considered before. If it didn't, then it made no sense to be working and leaving my son in someone else's care. I had to find another way.

So, I went back to NLP looking for some answers – I completed my full NLP Practitioner course and a coaching diploma and started coaching as much as I possibly could – early mornings before work, during my lunch break, in the evenings and at weekends. I adored it, and most importantly, the people I coached were experiencing some phenomenal results. I felt like I had finally found what I wanted to be when I grew up! I'd found my Zone of Genius.

Now the still small voice within shifted a gear – how could I find a way to build a business that enabled me to get paid to coach? How could I create a sustainable, profitable business of my own? And it was that voice that led me to the coaching conference I mentioned at the beginning of my story.

Since then I've grown, and stretched, and taken leaps way beyond the limits of my comfort zone. I struggled to keep up with myself at times – I felt I was free-falling at work and often got lost in the "how".

How could I leave my job? How could I run my own business? How could I find clients? How could I survive financially beyond the security of a regular salary? But beyond all of that was the pain of staying where I was – I felt I was "rusting from the inside out" and I had to take the risk to blossom.

On 1 November 2010 I launched what I thought would be a part-time business – one I would run alongside my academic career for a few years until it was stable enough for me to resign. On 8 November 2010 I was made redundant. The Universe had decided it was time for me to blossom; it was time for me to BELIEVE!

EXERCISES:

1. Find somewhere comfortable to sit.
Take a deep breath in through your nose and out through your mouth. Repeat, and each time you breath in, imagine your heart opening to accept everything good that you are breathing into your body (for example: self-belief, trust, love, acceptance, deserving, gratitude) and as you breath out, let go of anything that isn't serving you right now (for example: doubt, fear, confusion, staying small).

2. Use the breathing exercise above to ground yourself and connect with your heart.
Then find a mirror and look into your eyes. Deep into your eyes – the look you would give the person you adored most in the world. Say out loud "I am enough" –

how does that feel? What do you notice in your body? Is there another voice inside responding to what you have said? Say out loud again "I am enough" – again notice how you feel, where you feel it, and any words you hear in response to it. Repeat three more times – each time louder and from your heart, not from your head.

3. In times of fear use this exercise to face your fear: Ask yourself "What is it that I fear?" and "What could this fear be telling me that I need to heal?" Give yourself permission to sit with these questions and your answers to them. Accept where you are at and from that place of acceptance take one action that will move you forward.

Dr Michelle Clarke is an Authentic Success Mentor and Speaker who enables women to embrace all of who they REALLY are by giving them the tools and support to drop the "mask" that is holding them back from true success, abundance and feminine power.

BEAUTIFUL BEAMS OF HUMANITY
Sue Williams

You are a shining stream of sunlight,
A brilliant, beautiful, sight;
Shimmering, shifting, dancing;
Sparkling with pure delight.

Vital, vibrant essence of you; beaming,
Bursts bountifully through the gathering gloom,
Darting, dazzling energy lifts spirits; saggy,
Slumped, resigned within the room.

Engulfing each person present
with a glorious golden glow,
Warmth and love emerge;
until now buried deep below.
Boundless, bounteous, brilliance
of heart-warming humanity;
Enveloping all with sunny strength;
renewing their sanity.

BREAKDOWN TO BREAKTHROUGH
~ Babita Devi

"I am not what happened to me. I am what I choose to become."
Carl Gustav Jung

What is your calling and why does it matter? Is your life happening to you or through you? My name is Babita. I am a mother, a coach, and entrepreneur, but is this how I am defined?

For many years I believed that if I did what was necessary, I would be able to take myself to the next level. I thought that the more I had, the more I would be able to achieve. I just needed resources, time, energy, connections and clarity (hardly a small list) and then I could accomplish great things.

This belief didn't serve me well. I wasn't getting to where I wanted to be, instead I was swimming upstream. I started to see that 'how' I was showing up in my business was my limitation. Something had to change.

To understand the how, I had to go back to the beginning. So much of our thinking and our core beliefs are shaped by our experiences and the most profound of these are during our childhood.

Both my parents immigrated to the UK from India as children. My father arrived to look after his injured father, a World War 2 veteran, and my mother came to live with her aunt; both came in the hope of a prosperous future. Separation was a part of both of my parent's life, it was ingrained in so many of their experiences. When you move to a foreign country and you don't speak the language you can feel isolated from the world around you and even more determined to hold on to your core beliefs.

I saw my parents implement a simple equation - the harder you work, the more you earn. Their entrepreneurial spirit led to a multitude of business ventures, which continuously fell short of success.

Watching my parents go through this taught me a valuable lesson and the courage to pursue my own dreams, the valour to stay true to my calling and the might to push through the tough times that were to be part of my journey. They taught me the most valuable lesson of all, that there is no such thing as failure, only an opportunity to learn, and in some instances, pivot and adapt.

But there was an underlying theme that played out the whole time, they were immigrants, they were different, and they did not feel connected.

This question of fitting in influenced my early life too, starting with feeling the odd one out at school because English was not my first language. My elder sister and I were in the same year at school. Learning to live in the shadow of my older sibling was something that I became accustomed to, especially as I was the second girl born into a culture where boys and girls were treated very differently.

With a popular and bold older sister, I was never truly left out, just always on the periphery. At the time I did not realise this would continue to stay with me as I went through my adult life.

Fast forward to now, age 47. With 2 marriages and 2 beautiful daughters. It took me till my mid-forties to have the faith to start my own journey of truly finding myself. I had a longing to be alive, present and serve my purpose - something I continued to ignore until I had no choice. I had to break down before I could break through.

As I look back, I can say that my career has been marked with outward success. I have worked in high-level corporate jobs and founded a successful marketing business alongside coaching and lecturing. But all this was never enough.

I recall a specific moment in time when I realised that I was letting my life happen to me, like my life was playing on fast-forward. I desperately wanted to be present and to be a role model for my daughters; I knew I had so much more to offer. I realised that every part of my life needed to be in alignment for me to be truly successful in my business (beyond the financial side). If I wanted to leave a legacy and the world a better place, I needed to start showing up wanting to make that change happen.

Rewind to my teenage years. I left school knowing that I would never go to university, it was not an option as my parents were not able to afford to support me. So, I compromised my love affair with art for what some people would consider to be a more commercially viable career. I studied graphic design for two years and then went on to launch my marketing career, quickly rising the ladder and becoming a manager in my mid-twenties.

I learnt compromise early on, switching from desire and what was lighting me up to what the norm of society was, ticking the boxes of safety, security and working to provide. I don't regret any of this as I have truly enjoyed, and continue to enjoy marketing. It was and is the happy medium between a commercial focus and creativity, and this put me in good stead for what was to come.

Working my way up through the ranks, in jobs where I was mainly surrounded by men, I quickly realised that I needed a different stance. Looking at my world from the inside out was very different from how the outer world was seeing 'me'. I continued working in marketing and with every job, I set out to make a difference.

When I had the opportunity to move to Australia in 2004, I decided to set up my own marketing company called bStrategic. Fortunately, my reputation pulled me through and I didn't have to market myself much; my work came easily through word of mouth and recommendations.

After living in Australia for a couple of years I decided to move back to the UK. I considered myself lucky that I was able to move my business between continents and cities. However, the moves were becoming increasingly challenging for my older daughter who was 5 at the time.

Hopping between cities meant that she had to start a new school several times, a testing time for any child. The moving and the real-life challenges sparked my second business; a parent communication app called mySircles. It came from both my own personal need to support my children, but also the desire to help others as they manage the transition into parenthood and school life.

I had a deep desire to help take away some of the anxiety children and parents feel as they go through school, but also to share the celebrations through a connected parent community. I realised that as parents we need to strengthen our communication, so we can support our children through their growth and development.

Gone are the days when parents would just hang around at the school gate. Technology has started to play an important role in both parents' and children's lives for lots of reasons. I wanted to help parents use technology to enhance their child's journey through school by connecting with the school and other parents. I knew that the small ripples of communication would create waves and have a larger impact on the lives of our children and their future.

When I first began exploring the idea of creating an app to connect parents, I treated it like a pet project and made excuses to stop me moving forward with it, blaming the slow progress on being busy. It was then that the universe showed up to guide me; I was presented with a choice and I either had to decide to stay in my comfort zone and compromise what I truly wanted or take the plunge and sacrifice everything that was 'comfortable'.

The time to make this choice came when a large client asked me to take a full-time role. If I refused the offer, it would mean losing my consultancy contract with them. I walked away. This made space for mySircles to grow.

Now was the time, I had to step up!

I started on my journey of setting up a technology company. In June of 2015, I started to learn all that I could about the marketplace, talking to anyone that was prepared to help educate me; and people just appeared, willingly giving me their time.

Although exhilarating at first, this time is my life was extremely challenging. No matter how hard I worked, I just could not make headway. I found myself in a dark place. Better known as 'the breakdown.'

I have since learnt that this is part of the process that very few entrepreneurs manage to avoid. After having invested a large part of my personal savings, years of sacrificing a handsome salary that I had become accustomed to, I found myself in the darkness of self-doubt. I was broken and the thought of facing any more rejection, challenges or failures filled me with deep dread.

When you are in this broken place and there is nowhere else to go or hide, there is only one way out. As I began to peel back the layers of what was happening, I soon began to realise that I was my own limitation standing in my own way.

My beliefs, self-esteem and judgements were holding me back. The only thing stopping me was me.

I made the bold decision to look inside and do the inner work. No sooner had I put out to the universe that I was ready for the next step, my support team arrived. What took place next was nothing short of pure transformation. With help from my own coach, I learnt that the showing up isn't all that matters. It is the how!

I now have an amazing app that I am ready to take to the world. I know I can make a difference, my belief and all that I am is true through every action that I take. I can make a difference to the lives of children, by connecting parents and enhancing their child's journey through school. Before this could happen, I had to be that person; once that decision was made, everything else fell into place perfectly.

This is the same decision that also led to me funding a computer centre in the village that my parents are from in

India, teaching underprivileged children basic computing skills. I am thrilled with the impact it's having on the local children, the ripples it is creating. This is just the start, I will continue to help the future generation really find themselves, do the things that excite them and realise how they too can have an impact.

If you are reading this book, it won't come as a surprise that when we take that leap of faith, the universe has our back and is always ready to catch us. The only question we need to answer is how far are we prepared to fall before we decide to show up differently? How much of you will be broken, before you step up and break through?

What experience will it take for you to know that every contrasting situation is an opportunity for growth? Every emotion that is stirred serves to remind us whether we are in alignment or out of alignment. The journey of this transformation is a one-way street, once you discover yourself, you will never look back.

EXERCISES:

Here are some practical tips to help you flow downstream in your business, get back in touch with what lights you up and to help let the universe guide you to the change you are looking for.

Give yourself permission to enjoy the day today. Start by being grateful for all the positive things around you – no matter how small.

ACTION: Write down 5 things that you are grateful for. Spend time in the morning doing whatever raises your vibration and keeps you in a 'happy' place. Go for a walk, listen to music, sit in a café with your favourite book.

ACTION: Spend at least 30 minutes doing something you enjoy without feeling guilty.

Look at yourself in your business or place of work from the outside. What do you like about where you are and what don't you like?

ACTION: Make a list of what you do and don't like – don't stop until you have written everything down.

Take time to meditate. If you struggle and have too many thoughts in your head, go with a guided meditation. Ask specific and direct questions. See what surfaces. If nothing surfaces straight away, don't worry as you just need a little time. Keep an open mind.

ACTION: Write down anything that comes up.

Stay mindful for the rest of the day. What nudges are you getting? Are you being called to do something? Whatever it may be and however disconnected you might think it is... do it!

ACTION: Write down one thing that popped into your mind as an action and do this one thing.

Babita Devi is a mother, coach and entrepreneur. She set up bStrategic in 2004 – a marketing company helping organisations connect more effectively with their customers. In 2015, she created mySircles, an app to build stronger communities, again centred around connections.

She has also mentored marketing teams and more recently started coaching female business owners. Her 90-day transformation program is designed to help people that are looking to make a change from the inside out.

Babita's soul purpose is to help make a difference to the lives of others so they can step into their light.

CELEBRATION
Sue Williams

Too often we forget to celebrate.
We go about our tasks, move from one to the next,
Become irate, frazzled, suddenly vexed,
Perhaps it's because we left it too late to celebrate.

To achieve takes time. There is reason in the rhyme,
Rhyme in our reason.
Constant as the changing season,
Life moves on.
Little time to revisit, ponder on, how creative
Flow addresses, those intricacies, our successes.
Stand back, admire the view, as artist purveys
Oil fuelled hue. Gaze anew, in awe and wonder,
At the brush-strokes fine,
reflected shine of golden gown.
I dare you, smile, appreciate,
disown that jaundiced frown.

Celebrate with pride. Before you resurrect your easel,
Pick up your fork, garnish your glass;
"pop" goes the weasel!
Dance, rejoice, shout and sing,
invite your friends to join right in.
It's in the celebration of our gifts
that the wisest truly win!

CORNER SHOP TO WEST END: ONE WOMAN'S TALE OF SUCCESS THROUGH ADVERSITY
~ Buckso Dhillon-Woolley

"If my life is going to mean anything, I have to live it myself". - Rick Riordan

"They want you and need an answer as soon as possible."

These were the parting words of my agent, Lee Morgan.

It was November 2014 and my husband was in Argentina, living it up with his diplomat friend who he would visit often. I wondered what the time was in Argentina and could I 'phone a friend'?

I had twelve-year-old twins at home who I also had to consider before deciding whether to take the year-long contract Lee had just offered.

What was I to do? Surely it was a straight "yes, I'll take it," kind of answer?! So, why was I so torn?

With my husband over 7000 miles away, I had no one to talk through this life changing decision I had to make immediately. I sighed. Why did everything good always come at a price? This current decision should have been a no-brainer. Instead, it felt like a game of "would you rather". I should have been ecstatic and overjoyed at the fact I was now being handed a contract to appear on one of the most coveted stages in the world, and yet there I sat, lamenting ALL the changes I would incur as a result of saying that one positive word.

You see, I grew up as a middle kid in a first-generation Indian family of six children; one of five girls. I was the proverbial black sheep, the only one who had high-faluting dreams to be a singer/actor when I left school. I was ignorant of the fact that my parents were just trying to live from day to day and feed a family of eight, never mind humouring their wayward, slightly chubby, darker-skinned, middle daughter.

There were never any supportive words of encourage-ment or daydreamy chats about what I wanted to be when I grew up, and this was pretty much the norm for me thereafter. There were, however, many chiding remarks for thinking that I even stood a chance along with twenty thousand other wannabes who were all trying to make it. With hindsight, I now realise that my poor parents didn't have a clue how they could even begin to help their ambitious middle kid with her dreams and aspirations… and so, they didn't.

After leaving school, with no qualifications above a C grade, I was immediately informed that I would have to run my dad's new business in Derbyshire. It meant finishing up a brief stint working for a travel agency, which I loved. I found ways to enjoy my work. I enjoyed chatting to all the customers and hearing their stories of life and learning lots along the way.

This one chap named James really stuck out. He would regale stories of the West End and his time as an actor in London. I'd listen, totally enraptured by his tales of excitement and flamboyant behaviour in the 70s. Namely, him strutting down Carnaby Street in a Canary Yellow 3-piece suit! These conversations, I now realise, kept my embers of desire burning for the love of all things stage.

74

Nowadays, the words they would use for this are "affirmations" and "gratitude". You see, what I was doing back then was visualising all his antics with him, feeling the emotions attached to them and igniting the possibility that I might actually do this myself one day! How this would happen was never discussed, I just knew I was going to live this life one day.

We often become so wrapped up in how we are going to get from A to B, that we forget to feel into why we want something so badly. Although the term Law of Attraction is generally familiar now, having been around for a long time, back in the 1980s I didn't know the relevant term for it. With hindsight, it was the Law of Attraction that I was applying to my life back then.

Hearing James's stories led me to start making my own decisions. Regardless of whether or not I would get support from home, I knew I was going to act.

This brings us back to the start of my story. Did I go to London for 12 months? Did I leave my family behind to do this? Was it everything I hoped for and more? Yes, Yes, and No.

My decision caused changes in our lives that affected all of us, not just me. My husband had to switch from full-time to part-time work, which was a huge ask of him. I only saw the kids every Sunday afternoon, unless I was on annual leave from the show. I was living alone most of the time in a two-bed flat in London, which may sound like heaven initially but the novelty soon wore off when I was mugged at gunpoint three months into my stay.

After the show ended, I was diagnosed, with rheumatoid

arthritis as a "thank you for all your hard work Buckso," or that's how it felt! Next ensued months when I fell into a dark hole.

After I returned to Derbyshire and the family that I'd missed so desperately, folks would constantly ask if I'd loved my time performing in the West End. "Oh, I bet ya did!" they'd say. I could have shouted from the bottom of my now very sore lungs, that "No, I didn't love it down there!" Getting mugged, developing the auto-immune disease, losing precious time with my kids and husband; none of that was loveable. But I didn't say any of this. I just smiled and said: "Yeah, it was ace!"

That's what they wanted to hear. In fact, so did I. I didn't want to feel as if it had all been for nothing. It took me the best part of two years to eradicate the negativity I'd attached to that experience, even to the point of considering giving up the acting game.

I knew that somehow, I had to restore my self-belief. I needed to revisit my "daydreamer days" back in the shop and remind myself why I was still going to do this. I started to tackle all and any emotions I was going through, determined not to avoid anything that might come up. It was a hard time, but equally, so very healing and I am so grateful to those folks that came into my life and enabled me to release the shackles I'd put myself in.

Releasing involved energy work, self-realisation and raising the vibrations in my energy field through hands on healing.

Fact: we cannot and will not prosper to our full potential, if we continue to avoid that which we are resisting.

Today, I am very happy with the fact I decided to stay in the acting game.

I have also branched off to become a confidence and mindset mentor. I prefer to focus on the good that came out of my time in London, such as my friends, my networking connections, and most of all, a stronger relationship with my husband.

Yes, my dears, it was ALL worth it in the end.

EXERCISES AND DAILY PRACTICE:

This is a link to a lovely meditation piece on YouTube. I light incense and listen to it first thing in the morning around the house as part of my every day routine. You may want to try it when you first wake up. http://bit.ly/2D5ug7f

Read or listen to Napoleon Hill "Think and Grow Rich." I recommend that you listen to it multiple times and never stop listening to it, as you will always hear something new each and every time. YouTube has a free audio version - http://bit.ly/2TKCbg4

Whenever you're having a really good day and feel like you're on cloud 9 don't just "enjoy" it at the time. Use that moment to take you to the next level by putting on your favourite tune and dancing around the room, or sing at the top of your lungs like no one is listening. This will increase your vibrational frequency even more. Capitalise on the good days to keep the bad ones at bay; or at least appear less frequently!

Buckso Dhillon-Woolley is an Actor / Speaker / Voiceover / Presenter and Singer. She has achieved success through her own determination and tenacity, appearing in ALL the UK soaps (except the elusive Holby!); Unforgotten and The Tunnel, and a stint in the West End, culminating in her Disney film debut in 2019. A Confidence and Mindset Mentor, Buckso supports others to realise their ambition whether in their personal or business lives. She also teaches confidence to communicate to camera.

I SEE YOU
Sue Williams

I see you, women of the world.
I see your glory, feel your pain;
I sense your loss, celebrate your gains.
I sense your sadness, hidden joy,
I rejoice in the gifts you daily employ.

Join together, rise, sisters, rise;
Send fervent wishes soaring to the skies.
Realise your dreams, claim your power;
Appreciate every day, each emerging hour.

Empathy, care, freedom, fun;
Completing tasks that need to be done.
Thank the Lord for what you have:
Partners, friends, family, community,
With whom you connect, create true unity.

Rise as women, alongside men,
It's not a case of "us against them."
Hold the space, grasp the reigns,
Softly stroll down country lanes.
Own your inner, feminine gifts;
Create new meaning, life changing shifts.

Stand up and speak your authentic truth,
Silenced so cruelly in your youth.
Easing into grace and flow,
Allow your energy to expand and grow.
Sensitive, gentle, courageous, strong,

Within you, gratitude, joy, belong.

Regain your true essence, inner worth,
This is what will save the earth.
Allow past hurts to fade and die,
Claim your inner reason "why",

Achieving balance, grounded, real,
Allowed your own thoughts, desires to feel,
Nor your pain, your hurts conceal.
When with overwhelm, doubts you reel,
Look around, you're not alone,
For decades women have been coming home.

I see you, you are not alone,
I see you, as a woman, not a drone,
I see you, my Queen, reclaim your throne.

TURN UP THE LIGHTS
~ Helen Elizabeth Evans

"Your playing small doesn't serve the world.
There is nothing enlightened about shrinking
So that other people won't feel insecure around you."
Marianne Williamson from a letter to Oprah Winfrey,
published in "A Return to Love"

Have you ever lain in bed in the dark and looking across
the room you see a shadow, and the more you look at it
the more convinced you are it is something scary?

You tell yourself your eyes are just playing tricks on you
and it's nothing; but the more you try to make sense of it
the more you can feel your heart starting to race... just a
little.

Eventually you can't stand it, and you turn on the lights!
You discover your scary monster shadow is… your coat
and hat draped on the back of a chair. You laugh and turn
the lights off again, feeling really relieved!

That analogy really expresses so beautifully what I have
learned in my life, and I hope that my sharing the
following part of my story with you will save you the
years of resistance, angst and frustration I have put myself
through!

Do you procrastinate? Do you feel confused about where
you should focus your efforts? Are you unsure about

what you are really good at? Do you feel like the odd one out, struggling to find where you really fit in?

That was me… directionless, feeling stuck and severely lacking in any real self-belief. I was so desperate for my life to have meaning; for the effort I put into things to have some point…

I didn't start life like that. I was a real go-getter, confident and enthusiastic about exploring all life had to offer, but then each time life offered something that wasn't "great" in any form or fashion I lost a little enthusiasm, I lost confidence and my ability to know what I really wanted.

In fact, I ended up in a form of stasis, lost, just reacting to whatever came along in life rather than directing my life. I wanted to fit in, I wanted to belong and to be accepted and I learned to get these needs met by fulfilling other people's expectations. My image of myself developed from what other's reflected back at me, and I didn't love that image at all, so I found ways to hide out more and more, to avoid being seen, to avoid getting involved.

This would manifest in different ways:

I'd make excuses or create crises to give me reasons not to go to a social gathering or event, not to take someone up on an opportunity they'd offer me.

I'd spend my life apologising to people, so if someone said "I had a really bad day and this guy stole my parking space and now I've stayed in all day waiting for the electrician to turn up… etc." I'd find myself saying "I'm sorry" like it was my fault, like I somehow had to fix their day for them!

If someone complimented me on something, I'd dismiss it or give credit to someone else. One example was, if my husband and I had a dinner party and our guests said how much they'd loved the dessert I'd made I'd say "Yeah, it was okay, but wasn't the main meal Daniel made amazing?"

I always deflected attention away from me.

I'd take responsibility for everything as if it was all my fault rather than possibly being partly my fault, e.g. when my kids behaved badly, I thought it was my fault for not being a good enough parent, or if someone was rude to me, I'd think I'd done something to cause them to be rude to me.

I didn't know what I wanted. I had no vision for my life. I thought what everyone else wanted was more important than what I wanted. I felt undeserving.

Life was no fun, and I just didn't feel good enough. How miserable was that!

Seriously, if your life is currently like mine was in any way, then the only answer is to laugh out loud. How on earth do we let ourselves get into these states?

The metaphor that best describes what had happened to me is this one: if you put a frog in hot water it would jump right out, slightly scalded but fine, whereas if you put a frog in cold water and heat it really slowly it would just get sleepier, not realising its peril and die.

We often accept things that happen to us in life because on their own they are not that big a deal, but as we keep accepting these experiences that diminish us a little more each time, we don't realise the peril we are in until we are depressed and miserable, with a view of ourselves that is the equivalent of the scary monster we see in the dark in the corner of our room.

I would have moments of lucidity where I knew I wasn't happy but I had no idea how to change that, so blanked out what I was feeling and just got on with life, effectively allowing my self-worth to deteriorate further. I kept looking for ways to solve the problem my life seemed to be, and then felt more and more stuck because I didn't seem to be able to make any significant difference.

Then at 39, my daughter was born. I had wanted a daughter so badly and had some trouble conceiving her, so when she arrived a shift happened for me. I'd finally got what I really wanted. Now what? I had ticked all the expected boxes. I was happily married; I had a son and a daughter, a lovely home in Kensington (London), two gorgeous furry "people" (cats) and a successful property services business of my own. I no longer had anything to distract me from myself and my experience of myself.

This was the first step in my healing process, creating the space where I had no choice but to stare at the scary monster shadow I thought was really me, to really look at myself. Not a pleasant experience, but also not as bad as I expected!

I've learned that we need to look directly at what we perceive to be the worst version of ourselves and accept that version, realising we are just doing the best we can with the resources, the experiences and know-how we currently have. Accepting yourself and forgiving yourself for not being perfect, according to whatever undefined set of rules you hold in your subconscious, is usually the biggest and most profound step toward your healing. The second step was to find and accept my inner truth, and this happened through a few experiences.

The first was facing the reality of death, not my own, but a friend my age who should never have died but did. It was a shock to my system. I wanted her death to mean something; so, I chose to honour her by choosing to live differently, not to waste my life in the illusion of being stuck, depressed and feeling unworthy.

The second was discovering "The Last Lecture" by Randy Pausch on YouTube. Here was a man knowing he had little time to live and yet was living more fully than I ever had. Two things in particular stuck with me. He said "Walls are there so you can prove how much you want something" and "You need to decide if you are a Tigger or an Eeyore". How liberating to think like that! I have always been a Tigger. I am happy. I bounce. I had just forgotten. And walls? They'd never been an issue for me before. I'd always found a way around them in the past. I just needed reminding.

These two things, plus my openness to finding a different way, meant that I was in a different place when I re-read the quote made famous by and often wrongly attributed to Nelson Mandela, from Marianne Williamson's book "A Return to Love". Sometimes when we read something it doesn't do anything for us. We need to be in the right state to see and absorb the message in the words:

"Our deepest fear is not that we are inadequate.
Our deepest fear is that we are powerful beyond measure.
It is our light, not our darkness, that most frightens us."

Feeling not good enough was my illusion. It was my power that had always got me into "trouble" all my life, and I now viewed it as a bad part of myself because expressing it brought me pain. So, I tried to hide it. When you turn your power in on yourself by trying to cover it up it just eats you up inside and that can manifest as depression, self-loathing, anger, frustration or feeling stuck. Of course, as much as I tried to hide it, others sensed it anyway and so it still caused me grief because I was now coming across as incongruent…

Accepting I was powerful and could not change that was a massive relief. It did not make my problems with using my power go away, but just accepting that part of me that I struggled with so much was a huge leap forward.

In another part of the quote Marianne says:

"Your playing small doesn't serve the world.
There is nothing enlightened about shrinking
So that other people won't feel insecure around you."

This really hit home. It was exactly what I'd been doing all along. My big marshmallow heart thought I needed to diminish myself in order not to upset those around me. The reality is that if we all stay hidden in the shadows looking at ourselves and those around us as scary monsters because we can't see them properly in their diminished state, then we're all going to stay there forever. We need to turn up the lights and see ourselves for who we really are!

Marianne expresses it so beautifully:

"And as we let our light shine,
We unconsciously give other people permission to do the same.
As we are liberated from our own fear,
Our presence automatically liberates others."

The realisations that occurred in this process were the equivalent of taking my armour off and feeling very exposed but it brought about the third step in my healing process and that was to create a state of curiosity in my way of being with myself and the world around me. Being curious involves no judgement, just the act of noticing.

Taking the judgement out, letting the internal chatter say what it needed to and then letting it go, was transformational for me. I suddenly saw that no matter the situation, person or thing, it's all just perspective. It's how we perceive what happens to us in life that determines how we respond to it and thus the results we get.

We have a choice. We can change how we see things to change the results we get. For example, if you see a houseplant looking half dead you may throw it out, whereas if you see it as simply in need of some proper light and less water and take action in that way, you will give it back its life and delight in the difference you made. This is a simple analogy but you can apply it to anything.

My biggest shift came when I discovered fingerprint analysis, which had such a profound impact on me that I have now spent years becoming the UK's premier expert in it. Suffice to say it gave me the validation and clarity I needed to turn up the lights, and I trust that soon it will be standard for every person to have their fingerprints analysed and know their life purpose formula from childhood.

The result is that I'm so much happier with a life that has focus and is filled with meaning and purpose. I know what holds me back and how to work around it.

I've accepted I am a bridge between the metaphysical and the real worlds, here to show others how to step into their light, see themselves as the beautiful, gifted beings they are and then show them how to manifest their purpose in the everyday material world.

So, look at the worst version of yourself, accept it, forgive yourself for it and move on. It's just one perspective.

Stop resisting the part of you that calls to the best version of yourself and start believing and living it. It is your inner truth. Be curious. Maintain a non-judgemental approach to yourself and others, and then start treating yourself the way you'd treat the person you most love and value in the world! This will begin your process of turning up the lights…

EXERCISES:

Here are some of the techniques I use to shift my perspective and choose my experience of life:

1. A fun way to connect with yourself is to get a large A3 piece of paper and in the centre write "Who am I?" Use the spaces on the paper to write thoughts that come to mind. Don't judge them or shorten them, just write what comes into your head. This is for you, not anyone else.

The key is not to write as if you were journaling but to put thoughts on to the paper all over the place; although you might want to allocate areas, e.g. for the things you like less put them in the lower part of the page and the bits you like in the top half of the page.

You may be surprised by some of the things you write... Draw squiggles around those you want to highlight. Mine is on the wall as it is a great reference for me whenever I need to come back to myself and remind myself about whom I am. As you evolve you can update it and develop it. I love to draw pictures and symbols on mine too! Make it yours in whatever way you can.

2. We all have rubbish days and so it is important to have ways to move out of the feelings those days generate.

    One of the ways I do this is to have a "treasure box". It's a box I love, that has my name on it and is filled with all the things I accomplish, the beautiful notes and cards people send to me or any keepsakes that remind me of how much I am loved and appreciated, how much I have really achieved. On down days I pull out my treasure box and find myself smiling and laughing in no time!

3. A technique I developed as a teenager that really changed my whole experience of life was one where I created the person I wanted to be in my head, my

values, confidence, skills, self-belief, way of walking, attitude to life, etc.

Then I created a picture of a "suit" that I would imagine myself stepping into whenever I went out into the world. I acted as if I was that person while in my "suit", giving myself permission to go back to being me when alone, but in no time, I discovered I was that person I wanted to be, even at home…

Helen Elizabeth Evans, the Fingerprint Analyst, is the UK's premier life purpose expert, working with dynamic women in business that want clarity, direction and purpose so they can focus their time, energy and money in a meaningful way.

Explore further at http://www.hands-on-business.com

THE POOL...
Angela Durrant

I emptied myself of all that I knew I was as
I sat there in the silence.
I noticed instead of the emptiness I expected to feel,
there was a pool.
The pool invited me to look into it.
As I looked into it, I saw my reflection,
but it changed in appearance upon my looking.
Gone were the sad, tear-stained eyes,
the heavy heart and drawn features.
I steadied my gaze, looking deeper into this image.
The reflection I saw gave me not blackness but light.
This pool at the bottom of my very self,
offered to change me...
I thought I had come to the end of my very self,
only to find a new beginning.

It had taken all of me to let go, to lose what I thought
I had gained by all my hard work.
I found a courage there by that pool
at the bottom of my very self.
I found a pool of love.
A vast pool of love, that beckoned me to visit often.
It spoke to me of gazing deeply into love's reflection
and finding all that I had yearned for.
I experienced a new sense of completeness
at the bottom of my very self by that vast pool of love.
Not just in the doing,
but in the being.

As I reflected upon myself, I knew there was
nothing I could offer this love,
only my tear-stained, wretched self.
I let my "self" go. It wasn't rejected at all.
This pool of love seemed to envelop,
even relish taking the heaviness from my soul,
covering me until all I could see was
a depth with no end.
I pulled my "self" out quickly...
fearful of what it all could mean.
I had never allowed myself to go this deeply before.
Who would I become if I did?
Would I recognise my "self"?
I had rules! I had lived by them!
I understood them,
even if they didn't make me happy!

I gazed back into the pool. I thought.
As I stood between two lives,
I knew there was only one way to go.
I had just tasted such an all-embracing love
that I knew it made more sense than the fear...
I let go.
I sank deeply...
I cried...
I laughed...

Then I was back.
The pool; no longer in front of me.
Normality was everywhere, cars beeped, people yapped,
and I just stood.
I stood and looked at my hands and I touched my face.
I was still me; I hadn't changed at all!!
No wait...

There was a smell, a new smell, a fresh kind of
just washed linen kind of a smell that entered my nostrils.
Then I knew it... I knew what I must do.
I took a step forward, then another,
strength and vitality returning to my legs with every step.
I began to stride, then to run.
My legs and arms moved with a new purpose.
I stopped and breathed deeply of what felt like new air.
New birth.
Then I noticed something very strange...
I still felt the pool...
I felt it warm my soul.
I looked up, I looked forward....
and I smiled.

BIG HEART, BIG MYTH
~ *Julie Anne Hart*

"Life's challenges are not supposed to paralyse you; they're supposed to help you discover who you are." Bernice Johnson Reagan

To be able to write this I am truly grateful for my life's experiences and the insight and enlightenment they have given me, and as I accept life's entire journey with a loving heart, things continue to just get better.

It is so lovely to share our thoughts and experiences in order to heal on our path to wholeness.

I'm not going to tell you my whole life story simply because I want to get straight to the point. For most of my life, well 75% of it, I have felt worthless to be honest. I may not have identified it consciously, but in my actions, expectations and experiences it certainly showed itself!

Having spent over 15 years on a personal, professional and spiritual healing quest, learning many therapeutic practices that examine our childhood experiences, low self-esteem and low self-worth, I intuitively knew there was still something more than these issues at work.

Something so deeply rooted in my psyche that kept me so small, so frightened, so alone and almost totally unsociable. I was well out of alignment with the person I was starting to be aware of.

In the summer of 2000, I had a breakdown triggered by work-related stress. Although I was unaware of it at the time, it was actually a breakthrough on all levels: emotionally, physically and spiritually. I decided to take an alternative route with my health and well-being. I booked myself several natural healing sessions, which totally transformed my life. I began to have a sixth sense that was so strong I was hearing whispers and having visions, seeing and sensing like never before. I began a journey to find the truth about myself, and what a journey it has been!

My journey of truth has led me to numerous destinations and many spiritual teachers. In 2006, I was introduced to some of the ways of Native American people; the old and wise ways we have disconnected from, ways that made sense to me and felt right. This was the catalyst to a complete career change from social work to opening my own business, a small holistic shop, through to becoming an Intuitive Empowerment Coach.

I've always worked in community development and empowerment has been and still is my passion, only now I work in a very different way – I work with the guidance of a higher power.

As an intuitive teacher, coach and therapist I noticed in the clients that came to me a familiar thread that connected us all.

We were all very intuitive, gifted spiritual beings; yet no one owned it, felt it or acknowledged it. The creative development of the self was either maintained at a low level or destroyed, seldom reaching its full potential. So why was this?

Until now, I myself had never acknowledged the power of my intuition, I paid no attention to my thoughts and feelings and the message it was speaking through my whole body. I knew things that I wasn't aware of before, I was receiving direct information on all sorts of things; I was given guidance on work-related issues and I was aware of future events.

I can remember attending a meeting and knowing exactly what my boss was about to say. My inner wisdom had been activated and I have to say the power of direct communication with universal energy was very scary. I diminished it, hid away from it and remained blended with the wallpaper, unseen, unheard and in total denial of my truth.

My life experiences had been a mixture of abuse, co-dependency and FEAR, the most debilitating energy we create. I don't view myself as a victim and I don't feel like a victim because I am not one and neither is anyone else! So, here is my view on why we experience what we do.

Big Heart, Big Myth

Big-hearted intuitive people with a deep level of sensitivity, caring and compassion mostly want to be of service in a way that supports, heals and empowers others. Intuitive people have a unique energetic make-up consisting of universal energy; the source of love that runs through us. Often this uniqueness can be hard to acknowledge and handle.

If we look back in history, we see that those who show they are intuitive, gifted and special, as we all are, are often punished. The energy of fear that comes from being afraid of the magnificent ability of the self, shackles the body, mind and spirit and creates its own myth. A myth that tells its own story and a myth that creates its own EXPERIENCES, a myth that says we are not good enough.

If we can perceive that we create our experiences and choose the players in our self-created script to assist our highest healing and learning, then we can begin to awaken to the truth of what we have to learn about ourselves. What we create is what we think about ourselves and what we need to transform from the myth to the truth of who we really are.

So, is it really true your mother didn't love you, or your partner rejected you? Or is it part of your story that reinforces your inner beliefs about yourself. And so, your story begins and continues in the same mode of creation.

Little do we know, sense, feel or experience the truth of what is happening.

I am not releasing anyone of their responsibility here; we are all responsible for our own behaviour. What I am exploring is the correlation between the magnificent self and the self we destruct through self-created experiences that diminish our truth.

So, STOP and review your life. Are you really what you think you are? How do you feel about yourself right now? What would you like to change about yourself, your life?

There is nothing we cannot achieve. Our potential is totally unlimited and yet we do not see it or allow ourselves to feel it. The saddest part of all is not allowing ourselves to be our true selves.

Moving beyond our current illusion and into the reality of truth will take courage to heal our past experiences and move into energy of acceptance that will free us from our past perception. It takes strength to feel the emotions connected with our life experiences. Most of all, forgiveness and gratitude for the players in our story; those that hurt us the most often heal us the most.

My marriage was violent and abusive, but now I can thank my former husband. Through his mistreatment I ended my cycle of abusive relationships and used the experience to specialise in domestic abuse, working for 10 years in refuges and community development to assist women and children live abuse-free lives. My life experiences enabled me to work with greater understanding and insight.

It's time to begin with the truth that you are a magnificent creator, you are perfect as you are right now: unique, whole and complete. Dig deep and get clear on what's been happening and why. What program are you running?

The program I had been running was one of limitation of my potential coupled with shame that stopped me from receiving, and my message to myself was one of not being enough. But this was my myth, the way I kept myself safe and small. I had to wake up – life was calling me to become my truth. Waking up to the truth is never easy but the rewards are miracles in the making.

Vision Quest

Seeking enlightenment takes patience, time and commitment. Take a moment to ensure that you will not be disturbed. Light a candle in honour of yourself and allow yourself to question endless possibilities.

What if you invited your parents to play the roles they did to reinforce your myth about yourself? What if you did the same with your partner, and all relationships? What if they were just players on your stage, acting out your story so you could remain out of alignment with the truth of who you really are?

Sit comfortably and close your eyes and ask for the help and guidance you seek, allow the answers to flow through your inner knowing, listen to your thoughts and feelings – this is your intuition working through you and it will never let you down.

Who are you?

It is my belief that we are all so powerful, talented, loving and gifted that it makes it difficult to accept. We are love; it's the divine energy that runs through us. Love creates success and abundance on all levels and allows us to feel the bliss of harmonious emotion that will birth our dreams into our reality. And yet seldom do we allow our hearts to open on this level.

We create painful myths because we fear ourselves, our potential and our power. We fear others will fear us. Fear is a debilitating energy that only exists in the realms of our minds. The big pay-off to the big myth is that we can have all the primary gains to creating the myth, which are many things and all created out of fear: we get to stay the same, remain small and stay in the story that we do not want but which is familiar and comfortable.

Living the myth is time-limited because at some point not knowing or becoming your truth will be painful. It will be your soul telling you that you are more than what you think you are.

Stepping out, stepping up

I broke my cycle of illusory experiences through waking up to my inner truth and taking ownership of the self that creates everything inside me. I am fully responsible for everything I believe.

I began to look within to seek the answers from my inner being. The information I received back was amazing. I became more aware of my purpose, I started to feel and acknowledge my abilities and capabilities, my thoughts about myself began to change and so did my experiences. I view the people in my past experiences as helpers on life's journey to the truth about myself, and I thank and accept them for agreeing to play the role they did for the highest good of my learning. A difficult concept, but one that will accelerate your growth and quest to find the self.

Creating new wonderful experiences means loving yourself on a much higher level and opening your heart to allowing yourself to do so. To begin to achieve and receive all that your heart desires without the negative internal chatter inside your head. Stay out of your head and communicate with your heart, the core essence of you, the intuitive you, the higher self. It will always give you the true answer.

Big Heart, Big Purpose, Big Power

Having been closed to love for most of my life, I now understand why it's a miracle to be open to allow in all that the Universe wants to deliver and believe me, it is pure bliss.

We all have an amazing potential to love ourselves and each other. Allowing yourself to do this will move you to a higher vibration and a higher way of thinking and feeling that will free you from the shackles of your past.

Love will open up your intuition and the connection to your higher self, and will inspire you to realise your potential like never before. Opening my heart to more has allowed me to create my business and assist others with their purpose and potential.

Open your Big Heart, be your Big Purpose; step into your Big Power. We are here to make a difference so that we can all heal and be that which we are here to be. When you make a commitment to change the way you view your life and yourself, you have taken the first step of transformation to so much more. All you need is to be in the power of the moment and be ready to act on every opportunity that comes your way with trust and faith that your journey is being assisted each step of the way.

Stay focused on your dreams, and stay connected to the soul essence of you. Use all your senses to guide you, let your intuition speak through you. Your happiness is your guide to knowing you are walking your own sacred path.

EXERCISES:

And so, your journey begins right here, right now, with
the three easy processes listed below.

1. Open your heart to more love. This means acceptance
on all levels, with the main focus of acceptance being on
the self. This is a vital and an implicit element to seeing
the truth about you. Here there is no room for your
chattering negative mind to "sabotage things".

2. Make a list of all the things you feel about yourself.

Are these feelings positive, critical or judgemental? What
messages are these feelings giving you?

Look at your list again, shift your mind into neutral, think
nothing, move into your heart and ask yourself: is this
really my truth? Now write your truth from your
compassionate heart centre and compare and contrast it
with your myth. I did this many times. My mind was
telling me I wasn't good enough and my heart was telling
me to walk my path of beauty and shine. I had to allow
time to integrate my truth into my mind, body and spirit
by constantly affirming my truth.

3. Being Your Big Purpose is a mixture of your life
experiences, your passion to become all that you are and
your desire to achieve. Ask yourself what is it that I am
passionate about and why? What is my higher purpose,
what experience and wisdom have my life given me that I

can use to assist others for their highest good? Listen to your higher self, the intuitive part of you, and it will always give you the answer.

We all have an intuitive higher self to connect with. To do this you will need to calm the mind and open up your creative imagination and allow yourself to vision. Take some time where you will not be disturbed and close your eyes. Vision the self without self-created limitations, judgements or internal criticism and notice all your gifts, talents and skills. Really acknowledge YOU, and then write down how this differs from how you have viewed yourself in the past. Now stretch into the new concept of who you are.

As an Intuitive Empowerment Consultant, I feel blessed to be assisting so many people open their heart to their purpose, potential and intuitive power. I do believe that we have to return to our truth to make a bigger difference to ourselves, our families, future generations and to those that cross our path in need of our love, guidance and wisdom. In doing so, we create beauty and peace.

Julie Anne Hart is an Intuitive Empowerment Consultant specialising in Purpose, Potential and Prosperity.

You can contact her at www.julieannehart.com

CELEBRATING YOU
Sue Williams

Celebrating you, who you really are,
Every little blemish, hurt, cut and scar,
Women, you have travelled, so very, very, far,
Learned there is no need, to discard and burn your bra!

You have within you, everything you need;
Tenacity and talent, ability to breed.
Nurture, and love, every-one you feed;
Not forgetting yourself, receive, do not concede.

Celebrate your mothers, remember who you are,
Often, they could not drive their own car.
Travesties, injustice, resentment buried deep,
Gather all together, throw them in a heap.

Burn them on the brazier, chuck them on the fire,
You are a woman, stand in your power.
Watch old hurts smoulder, flames leap higher and higher.
You alone can claim your yearning heart's desire.

You are not an effigy, a plastic Barbie doll,
Don't deserve to be blackened by a troll,
Playing cards; you always come up trumps.
Don't let lewd comments drag you down into the dumps.

Talent, caring, creativity; yes, you also have a bust,
But not intended solely, as the subject of lust.
You can choose the outcome, you can sow the seed,
Yours is the decision, whether or not to conceive.

You can do the shopping, you can push the pram,
But only when you say; "this is not solely who I am".
I am a human being, whole in my own right,
I claim the facility for some well-deserved respite".

I fight my own battles, good as any man,
My choice of weapons, not just pots and pans.
I use wit and wisdom, anger when it's due,
I stand up, I count, just as much as you.

I can be a tomboy, or a "girlie girl",
I decide whether or not my hair will curl,
If colours, make-up, lipstick, I duly choose,
I can decide whether or not they match my shoes!

I am an intellectual, I am unique,
I have a voice; I stand up and speak.
I am understanding, I am not a sham,
I am a lady, yet, sometimes a "Madame"

Ladies, we are rising; no longer considered a crime,
It is not surprising, finally, it's our time!

REDISCOVERING THE REAL ME
Lynda Holt

"Use your effort and energy wisely, focus on who you want to be rather than who you think you can't be." Lynda Holt

We all have a story; it's made from what we choose to believe, our values and our habits. In our minds the story defines who we are and who we are not. It is this story we "show and tell" others about ourselves.

So why is it that so many people define themselves by who they are not and what they cannot do, instead of opening themselves up to the endless possibilities created by believing in what they can do, or even what they might be able to do?

For anyone who has read more than a few self-help books – and I've read a lot! – this whole positivity, self-belief thing seems obvious in theory; but perhaps not quite so easy in practice.

I believe there are some things that happen to us along our journey through life, often at quite a tender age, which either encourage us or stop us from being positive about ourselves. They are the things that re-calibrate what and how we measure our worth or success. They often start with other people's reactions to our behaviour, successes and failures. How we process these reactions can either support or undermine our opinion of ourselves.

I believe we put far too much credence on these perceptions because most of the time they say more about the other person's belief about themselves than they do about us. We let ourselves be moulded by these views and often change how we show up in the world in order to fit the role we think we play.

I'd like to illustrate what I mean by sharing my story. Like so many other people's stories there is no single life-changing event or evangelical inspiration that set the course of my world. Instead there were a series of life-changing actions, most of which I didn't realise were significant at the time.

So here goes. I was a pretty little thing with blond ringlets and chatty nature who delighted local adults with cute antics. This instilled in me a strong belief that people react well to me, I'm popular, interesting and funny. I can get people to do what I want if I work at it, and even better I can do or be whoever I want to be because they love me. Of course, as a toddler and pre-schooler I didn't process my belief in that way; that was just how it was. Therefore, the truth I believe about myself is – I can do anything I put my mind to.

So, I start school and the story continues: that vivacious, no outrageous, little girl has all the local boys eating out of her hand, running around, doing chores, carrying her PE bag, pumping up bike tyres, etc. Boy did I know how to work the charm! It worked because I believed that this is who I am and the boys enjoyed my company. We laughed, had fun, did all the things kids do, and because I felt good about me, I helped them feel good about themselves too.

That is how I thought life should be; that is what I believed we were worth. When any of my friends had a problem or felt unhappy, they came and talked to me – I didn't know why then, I just felt glad they did and that I could make them feel better.

Then something strange happened. The outrageous little girl turned into a gawky, self-conscious teenager. I moved to secondary school away from my village friends, I started to worry much more about what others thought, about fitting in, and I forgot to be myself. Expectations others placed on me – parents, teachers and let's not forget friends and peers, started to become my compass.

I began to question what I believed about myself, whether I was as good, as pretty, or as interesting as others and so on.

This is when the "I can'ts" start to define who you think you are. For example, "I can't sing, I can't do maths; I can't talk to boys" – whatever fits. Guess what, these "I can'ts" soon start to shape your life. Most of us stay in the place where we think we can because we don't want to feel exposed, we don't want to fail and often we don't want to fall short of others' expectations of us.

What about what we believe of ourselves? Well, that shrinks too. Certainly, it did in my case. So much so, that by the time I'd gone to college, got a career, bought a house had a baby and all that stuff we call life, I'd kind of forgotten who I was.

Sure, I had a great life, a lovely family, I had lots of friends, (especially ones who needed help) and was very successful in others' eyes. I had a good career in the NHS, where I had started as a nurse and progressed to someone holding national strategic positions, but deep down I knew there was more; more to give, more to be.

I also knew that the person I had become; the gawky teenager, the one who measured herself by others' happiness, who tried to please everyone, who fitted in with what was happening, and who quietly worked round obstacles and objections, while worrying about upsetting people; would not be the person to get more.

So, I came to a moment of decision – do I continue along this safe path or do I play a bigger game? Thankfully I rediscovered some of that outrageous little girl – the one who believed that if you want something you can have it; you just have to work out how to get whatever "it" is. In my case it was freedom, my own business, a break from the 15-year NHS career I'd once coveted.

At the time, of course, I didn't know this was what was happening; at the time I just thought I'd leverage my contacts and expertise and become a development

111

consultant. Business was great, I quickly got to know the high-profile people in my industry, collected a team of skilled people to work with and put myself in places where the clients I wanted would find me. Many seemingly small actions resulted in a lot of new opportunities and a whole different life to my NHS career. Definitely some traces of that outrageous little girl at work there!

Gradually I got more confident at both identifying and promoting the things I most enjoy; and funnily enough these are the same as the ones I am best at. My real satisfaction comes from helping people to see what they can do or be, whatever it is that's important to them. Just like I did with my friends when I was little; just as I'd done throughout my life for family, friends and colleagues – often thinking they only talked to me because I listen, and not seeing the real value I gave – which was to help people see their potential and to get out of their own way.

It took me a while to realise that success is about self-belief, drive and passion; not just skill, resources, and contacts – although these help enormously. Part of the reason it took me a time to realise this was because that self-conscious teenager got in the way. She would say "Who'd believe you? If it's that easy why doesn't everybody do it – silly?"

You know the kind of self-talk that knocks you off course before you even start. So, my first job was to sort myself out. After all, there was plenty of evidence to support my success, plenty of people wanting to work with me, and plenty of friends seeking my counsel – even though I only helped them see the answers they already had.

I say to people I am very lucky; I have exactly the business I want now, helping others to get out of their own way. I work with a great team and consistently meet fabulous, inspiring people. I believe that I am really lucky, not because of the business I created, but because I found myself again, I learned to believe in my gifts for the world and the value they bring. I went back to basics, examined what I believed about myself and asked two questions: Is this true? Does it serve me?

From here I reassessed a few beliefs based on my own evidence, the impact I had on people, the difference I made, not just the way I interpreted their response in the moment. I then got brave and decided not to settle for less than I could contribute – this bit is a work in progress, as there is always more we can do and be.

We have a choice in life, all of us do. We can choose to settle for where we are and let others define our destiny, or we can choose to define our own, little action by little action. By engaging with the real you, your passions and the things you were put on this world to give, you will find an authenticity which is easy to believe in.

You will discover that self-doubt slips away, you will find that small success after small success mitigates the times things don't go to plan, gives you the strength to deal with self-doubt and the power to keep moving forward, discovering more and more of the things you can do and can be.

How do I do it – well that's the easy bit – I found that outrageous little girl in me, the one who identifies what she wants and takes action to get it.

I hope you like my story and more importantly, I hope it makes you think about your story, who you are, what you want and who's running your life.

EXERCISES:

1. Spend some time thinking about how you define yourself, write it down or draw your vision – however you like.

Examine your beliefs about yourself and how you show up right now and ask:

Is this true?
Does it serve me?

Take out what is not true and what does not serve you currently, and then examine what is left.

2. Now imagine the best version of yourself, the one you've felt proud of, laughed with and enjoyed just being.

What are the characteristics, behaviours and beliefs of your best self?

Write or draw these and imagine how your life would be if this person showed up every day.

3. Identify what this person – your best self – is good at. What do they like doing, reading about; talking about? What do people seek this person's help with?

In these answers lie your gifts to the world. Try them for fit, and if you like them make them part of who you are and what you do.

Lynda Holt is the founder of Brave Scene, a community for ambitious business owners, and Brave CoWork. She works with business owners and leaders on courage, connection and growth. She is also a speaker and author of *"Get Out of Your Own Way"*.

Contact Lynda at www.lyndaholt.co.uk

I INTEND TO LIVE OUT MY PURPOSE
BEING HAPPILY GRANDIOSE
~ *Sarah Klugman*

The book bound by sadness, is reaching its end
It's a one-off edition, no sequels to be penned
Held safe, spine to spine, it has really been my mate
It has taught me it's wise, not to know my own fate

There are many, many chapters, all charting the course
Of a heart-broken woman, getting back on her horse
Tear stained pages, still hold their print well
And on reading them back, I am eased from my shell

My repetitive mantras, all laced with emotion
Held me responsible to myself and have set me in motion
I turned, facing my fear and caught my own eye
Recognising limitations, were what made me shy

Allowance. Allowing. We are designed to be our best
By letting go of control and letting life do the rest
It's okay not to know, it's okay to have joy
It's fantastic knowing I'm everything but the boy

The final pages of resolution, all fill up with light
The potential and possibilities, revealed in plain sight
It is now and forever; the door is open and won't close
I intend to live out my purpose, being happily grandiose.

LIVING THE AUSTRALIAN DREAM
~ *Elizabeth James*

"Be mindful. Be flexible. Believe!" Elizabeth James

Several years ago, my husband and I first discussed the idea of emigrating from the UK to Australia. Today, 25 November 2012, I spent the day on a beautiful Australian beach, enjoying life with my young daughter. We've been in Adelaide, South Australia, for six weeks – and, so far, we love it here.

Now, I'm not saying that getting to this point was in any way easy... but... all the planning, hard work and expense has most definitely been worth it.

Here's just one part of the story of how I came to be here today, living The Australian dream

During 2009 we spent four glorious weeks exploring various Australian cities. We came with open hearts and minds, and we absolutely knew within just two days of arriving that we'd be setting the emigration ball rolling upon our return to the UK.

During our "reccie" our goal was to live like Aussies. We rented typical suburban housing in areas we'd realistically consider living. We hired cars, and shopped in local supermarkets. I collected receipts, newspapers, housing sale and rental listings – anything I could get my hands on – and I kept a journal, detailing the entire trip, as research.

117

It was a very definite decision to bring our daughter into the world and give her several precious years with close family before we would ever emigrate. It also felt important to relocate before she became old enough to experience the heartache of separation. We knew it would be a bitter pill for all, but it seemed sweeter to the alternative of her never having that close time with family – and they with her.

Our girl was two-and-a-half years old when we left the UK. Of course, it had been heart-wrenching watching her grow closer and closer to her family, all the while knowing that they would soon be physically separated. However, special bonds were formed, and we all knew that we were paving solid foundations for the future. We continue to feel blessed by a supportive network of family and friends and I shall be eternally grateful for their unwavering encouragement and composure.

Knowing that the visa application process would take roughly 18 months we started proceedings when our daughter was six months old. My husband would be the main applicant as a Systems Administrator in Information Technology. We went through the full process of gaining points recognition before lodging the main visa application. We were to receive South Australian state sponsorship and permanent residency visas after only three months of submitting the main application.

My personal evolution
Maternity leave had afforded me the long-awaited

opportunity of completing several complementary therapy practitioner training programmes with a local holistic training college. In addition, I attended a weekly spiritual development program, and joined any spiritual and wellness workshops I could fit in.

I distinctly remember repeatedly announcing to fellow attendees that I was only attending all of these classes out of personal interest; that I wasn't a practising therapist, and neither did I ever intend being one!

It only took me a very short while, however, to realise that my exposure to the teachings and experiences was profoundly changing my life. My perceptions and beliefs were changing, along with my overall health and well-being as I made positive life changes. The realisation of my previous lack of self-worth was a particularly potent moment. I was learning and growing. I was changing. I was evolving.

My spiritual journey had begun, and I went on to complete training in Crystal and Colour Therapy, EFT, Sekhem, Reiki, Angelic Reiki, Past Life Regression Therapy, Numerology, Meditation Teaching and First Aid. I also achieved an ITEC-accredited Level 3 Diploma in Anatomy, Physiology and Pathology.

The college became my second home – a safe haven for personal discovery and development. As my knowledge and awareness increased, I began carrying out my case study treatments in order to complete my qualifications.

119

Working with clients away from the college brought the realisation of the responsibility involved. I instantly decided to become a therapist. I committed myself to completing the 100+ required case study treatment sessions. The feedback was immense! Now I was affecting the course of the lives of others. I knew I was helping.

Towards the end of my maternity leave, employer and childcare issues forced me to decide between returning to my previously well-paid management position – or not. Knowing that I would be sapped dry on every level if I returned, I handed in my notice. It was one of the most terrifying and yet liberating things I've ever done.

I crunched – and re-crunched – the figures before submitting my resignation. I had worked as a self-employed web and graphic designer for several years alongside my full-time position as a department manager for a global legal training provider.

I had regular private clients, but would they bring in enough financially?! I took up a part-time position at the college in order to ensure financial security. I committed to raising my daughter, organising the emigration, and my re-training.

I know now that I could never return to a desk job and would advise anyone to be brave and take that leap of faith as I did. Obviously try to ensure financial security beforehand – I'd spent seven years establishing a solid client base for my business before relying on the income from it in any way. Having said this, there was still that leap of faith and we can never really know what the future will hold.

Believing in magic, and manifesting
Shortly after submitting our visa applications, in October 2011, I attended a combined numerology and tarot reading. I had no idea what to expect, and I asked for guidance on the whole Australian dream. It was an insightful reading into my personality, with guidance on my needs for the upcoming year, all based upon my numerology.

The 12-month tarot spread was presented as "things to be aware of". A celebration was indicated for January 2012. I explained that this was when we were hoping for our visa grant decision, and that I already knew it was going to be a positive outcome.

This was the first time I realised that I had never doubted we really would make it to Australia. I realised that I had total belief that we would achieve our dream. I was manifesting it.

The reader encouraged me to move to Australia sooner rather than later – preferably during the summer. I explained that we were attending a wedding in July and that I wouldn't consider leaving before my mother's 60th birthday in September. I was advised that if we didn't move by October 2012 then we probably never would.

Inevitably, in the January we were granted our visas and I set about planning the big move for the relatively small window of late September. This followed the guidance I'd received, and also fitted perfectly with rental availability and a temperature change in South Australia. We would arrive in Spring.

As 2012 progressed it became clear that this was a pivotal year in my life. By now I was fully aware of the innate power of intention and manifestation. I knew that I would be dishonouring myself – including everything that I had become, and all who had supported me – if I were to walk away from the spiritually conscious life I had been building. In 2012 I consciously laid the foundations for mine and my family's future. I paved the way towards the life I wanted. People tell me I'm brave for quitting a well-paid, full-time job, re-training and moving my family across to the other side of the world. I've never felt brave. It never frightened me. It was a natural evolution.

Embracing change and being in the flow
As I developed spiritually, I became increasingly aware of "being in the flow". I was noticing more and more synchronicities around all I did. These little reassurances continue to help me know that I am on the right track.

We didn't enter into the decision to emigrate lightly, and I never underestimated my commitment to re-training – and doing so at the same time as emigrating! I have a "can do" attitude and face challenges head on. The downside of this is that I can push myself too hard and I try to move mountains on my own. The flipside is that I had the necessary determination and drive to make my dreams a reality. It is time to learn how to flow somewhere along the middle road.

I know I'm where I need to be, at just the right time. And that I'm doing exactly what I need to be doing. I embrace the learning and growth opportunities in every situation – of course, not always at the same time! This same scenario also applies to us all.

I believe that change is a good thing. Without it, how else will we ever grow?! Above all I have faith in myself. I acknowledge that yes, at this point I'm feeling weary – physically, emotionally and mentally. I've bordered on exhaustion to get where I am now. We only landed 6 weeks ago and it's been a long hard slog to get here. I acknowledge these consequences are the result of my own decisions.

I've driven how this journey has unfolded thus far. I own that. And having said that, I also know that I have a choice on how I move forward NOW. I choose health and well-being – on all levels - and I allow this to unfold.

I encourage you to consider that when things seem to be "going wrong", that this is merely your perception of the situation. You ARE in control – you control your reactions. Maybe sit and think about this: how have you allowed events and the actions of others to affect your feelings today?

Please allow me to share some moments from my journey, which I hope you'll find inspirational...

Selling our home in the UK
We left advertising our UK house for sale until far too late. The house had been on the market for ten weeks and we were getting close to leaving the UK. We'd already reduced the price and had no solid offers, despite a steady stream of viewings and positive feedback. Tensions were naturally fraught – we really wanted to sell before leaving the UK. We were starting to panic that the house wouldn't sell and had started arrangements to let it out instead.

A friend reminded me to manifest my purchasers, so I began focusing on picturing the people I wanted to buy our house – I detailed them right down to their age, family status, personalities, etc. I set the intention that these people would come along and buy our house for the right amount before we left the UK. As I greeted the next viewing couple at the door, we exchanged smiles – I instantly knew they were our purchasers, and of course they were.

I had also blessed our house the evening before that final viewing. We'd spent so many hours rushing around preparing for viewings – seemingly all for nothing – and we'd started to curse at the house. We were venting thoughts like how we needed to "get rid of the house" and "what else can this place throw at us". The evening before the final viewing I sat and realised that we'd been spouting out negative energy all over the house. Why would anyone want to buy a house which had all those low vibes floating around!?

I set my intention that I would fill the house with love. I placed rose quartz crystals around the house – purchased just days before from Chalice Well in Glastonbury (said to be the World Heart Centre). I used sound to energetically cleanse each room with my singing bowl and lit candles for ritual. I thanked the house for being a home to us. I acknowledged how we'd been happy there, and that house was all our daughter had known. I explained that we were ready to leave and I asked for help, explaining that I would find lovely new residents to also be happy there.

Now you may think me crazy in talking to a house! To me, I was respecting and honouring another step along my journey. And it worked didn't it?!

Securing the Australian house

One of the most exhausting challenges upon arrival in Australia was securing housing. It was important to set solid foundations and the house was key. I was researching until 3 a.m. most evenings. I was tired and this had been going on for weeks. Days were spent exploring suburbs and viewing countless properties. Each viewing gifted a new realisation; something we didn't want, or something we now knew we should be looking for in an Australian home. As a result of this, the search parameters changed each evening. It felt never-ending.

My husband was offered a job on a Thursday and was due to start work the following Tuesday. At that point we'd found four houses that we were reasonably happy with, although each one involved a compromise of some sort. I'd not given up on finding what we were looking for but we'd decided to make a final decision by the Monday before my husband started work. Enough was enough. We needed stability.

On the Friday I'd scheduled a meeting with a kindergarten principal at 10 a.m. I had been researching until past 4 a.m. the evening before and was exhausted. When the alarm went off my first instinct was to throw it through the window! I considered cancelling the meeting and talked myself in and back out of doing so twice. I decided to keep the appointment at the last minute.

The meeting was very successful – the centre is wonderful and my daughter is now happily attending playgroup there.

During the meeting I mentioned the terrible time we were having trying to find the right home. The principal promptly called in one of the teachers, who I discovered was looking to rent out her house. The house had the number of bedrooms we'd been looking for, plus full solar power and a swimming pool. It ticked the boxes!

Assuming it was going to be way over budget, I tentatively asked about the weekly rent and was delighted to discover that it was actually below budget.

126

Furthermore, the house was located directly across the road from the kindergarten and we were invited for an instant viewing.

The house overlooks a beautiful natural gorge and the surrounding gum trees are regularly host to a number of koalas and kookaburras. There is a large decked balcony to the rear, direct gated access to the gorge, windows lining the entire rear of the property, a large spa bath, dressing room, large rumpus room, and a well-established lemon tree – which I loved! It exceeded expectations.

The house hadn't yet been advertised, and we were the only ones to view. We moved in before the New Year. Right time... right place, and/or divine flow? What's the difference?!

EXERCISES:

1: Set goals and do something about working towards them

Reach for your dreams and realise what a powerful manifestor you truly are. Sit and meditate (mindfully reflect) upon your life. Where are you heading? How do you WANT your life to be? What's stopping you, really? Motivation comes from the satisfaction of ticking off a goal, so first spend time thinking about what your goals actually are. Break your goals down into smaller, and more manageable tasks. Try not to impose strict deadlines, although assigning a timescale is a great idea so that you're accountable for taking action.

Write your goals down – a mounted vision board is a great way to help with ongoing focus. Be sure to use colour energy and symbolism for added effect – i.e. green for growth, red for courage and drive, yellow for confidence.

Take daily steps towards achieving your goals and remember that no matter how large or small these steps may feel to you; they're still steps in the right direction.

You won't go anywhere if you stand still.

2: Have a contingency plan, be flexible, and expect change

Circumstances change, and so too should your plans. Don't get too hung up on this and try to remember that YOU are the only one who gets to decide how YOU are feeling in any one moment. If you allow hurdles to stress you out then that's exactly how you'll feel – stressed.

Consider seeing challenges as welcome opportunities to reassess your plan. We learn and grow through these moments.

It's wise to have a Plan B – maybe even have Plans C and D on standby. By spending time thinking of alternative scenarios in your "perfect" plan, you'll be better prepared for when things change – which they inevitably will.

3: Be true to yourself and believe

Above all, remain true to yourself in all choices. Don't ever allow yourself to become someone you're not. You'll feel this in your belly – this is your gauge for knowing when something is out of alignment. Slow down, listen.

Be honest with yourself.

It's fruitless, and actually quite damaging, to sacrifice your own wants and needs for the sake of another's priorities or, worse still, in the event of feeling repressed.

Suppression leads to dis-ease – FACT.

We're each on this planet, at this time, for a purpose. It really does only take one person to bring about change. Be conscious of your choices; your thoughts, words, and actions. We've each chosen to be here. Now choose to be present.

We each have our own path to follow and gifts to share. You really are perfectly you. Own that.

Thank you for reading.

Elizabeth James is a tutor and holistic practitioner who is following her dreams in the Adelaide foothills, South Australia. Elizabeth runs a thriving practice along with weekly mindful meditation classes and a range of monthly support and spiritual development circles and workshops.

Elizabeth sculpts and creates art, and also runs various aged care support and wellness programs across the local council area. Elizabeth actively maintains an online Facebook community page at www.facebook.com/lotusstartherapies and offers free weekly mini readings and online support and sharing.

You can follow her work at www.lotusstar.com.au

WHERE DO I GO FROM HERE?
Cheryl Bass – *Founder of I Am Woman*

Where do you go next,
when your throat can't find words
your eyes only find tears
and you feel nothing?

You gaze around the room, seeking some reassurance
that life after all is worth living,
even though just being here is laced with sadness.

A thought flickers through and ricochets
around the head, my head.

I forget that this pain belongs just to me,
no one realises the depth of this depression.

Like a little girl I beg to find
something to look forward to
but then feel the pain of anxiety
that rises up inside me because
where there is false hope there is disappointment.

A pit of dough fills my stomach
that pushes up to release a swallow
the same swallow that just releases
more tears to my eyes, nothingness to my ears.
Another evening alone in myself, so very alone in myself
When will someone step in me,
with me,
to help me
take that first step from here.

COMING HOME

Cheryl Bass — *Founder of I Am Woman*

Journeys start, journeys end and
in my heart I've found my friend.
No more searching, no more waiting,
no more denying I already have it all.

Why do we search waiting for outside confirmation,
outside love, outside happiness?
When all the time inside we can unwrap
our most beautiful gift to ourselves, love.

Coming home to me has been
a terrifying journey in accepting no one is coming,
because they were here all the time,
all the time.

That person that kept me safe, kept me whole, kept me alive.
She held me when I cried, wiped my tears of pain away and
helped me get up when no strength was present.
She was always at home waiting to love me, hold me and listen.

No more outside confirmation that this me is ok;
just coming home to me and being perfectly me.
Because I know her so well,
her living dreams and her living hell.

Whatever she wants it's mine to deny or mine to give,
but in this body and in this soul, it's my pleasure to live.

Family, friends and lovers will come and go,
but I will always be here with myself travelling on,
always coming home.

CHOOSE TO CHANGE
~ *Helen Killeen*

"The most beautiful people we have known are those who have known defeat, known suffering, known struggle, known loss, and have found their way out of these depths. These persons have an appreciation, sensitivity and an understanding of life that fills them with compassion, gentleness, and a deep loving concern. Beautiful people do not just happen." Elisabeth Kübler-Ross

Some people don't have the best start in life but I truly believe that anyone can make a choice to change. My choice to change helped me overcome a past where I had experienced many difficult challenges that for a long time had a very adverse impact on my life. This damaging impact caused me to suffer great depression, stress, anxiety, panic attacks and bad thoughts about life and whether to continue with it or not. I once wrote this very negative statement:

No one knows the horrible images that go through my mind that I have to battle with every day. The depression that consumes me which I have to crawl out of, the anger inside of me that I have to fight with, the loneliness that kills my soul, the anxiety that eats away at me and the constant pain in my heart that I have to endure. I feel the devil pursues me.

How destructive does that sound! No wonder I was such an emotional wreck all the time, crying at everything, worrying about everything and feeling guilty over everything. I didn't realise it at the time, but because I was dwelling so much on the bad things that had happened to me, I was the one bringing a whole lot more negativity into my life.

This may sound strange to some people but having read the book 'The Secret' I soon came to realise that my negative thought patterns were attracting many more negative situations and bad feelings about myself.

But how did I get to this point?

Well a lot of it was to do with things that I had been through in my past that I had not yet dealt with; the emotions of what I had been through were building up inside my mind and starting to drive me insane. My mind was a battlefield. Not dealing with these emotions was stopping me from getting the life I wanted and deserved.

By dealing with it, I mean, coming out, talking to people about what happened and about how I was feeling and finding a way of coming to peace with it all.

It took one person to really believe in me and to make me see that I had to deal with these things in order to change the course of my life. I am truly grateful to my wonderful friend Lisa Incorvaia for coming into my life and making me believe that I could finally find peace in my mind. It felt like I had been waiting for her for so long and I feel that God had sent her to me.

The reason I feel this way was because sitting at home one day after calling in sick at work due to the depression I was feeling I said out loud 'please help me God'. The very next moment I had an email from this lovely Lisa asking how I was and saying that God had put me in her heart that day. Very strange isn't it. I never really believed in God before this point and cursed him and blamed him a lot for all the terrible things that I had experienced.

So, I will tell you about some of what I experienced in my life, how I stopped playing the victim and chose instead to use my experiences to help others choose to change, and demonstrate that you CAN choose to change. I'm sorry if you find some of this upsetting and shocking.

From the age of 10, I was abused by someone (and I want to point out that it was not by a close relative, but someone who happened to be in my family's life until I was 16). This went on for a long time. Then at the age of 13 I watched my dad die of cancer. After my dad died, I then took on the role of carer for my mum and the responsibility for the house. I came from a family of three brothers and one sister who were all much older than me, so they had their own lives and children to support.

As soon as I started secondary school, I started drinking a lot of alcohol, which I think helped with the pain of what I was going through. I was quite a quiet and shy girl, so I didn't really speak much about how I felt or talk to anyone about what was happening to me. I was always too concerned about everyone else's feelings and not upsetting anyone and trying to make everyone happy, never really thinking about myself. For a long time, I felt that no one really cared about me.

I didn't do very well at school, leaving with just one GCSE grade C in Art, and again this was something for me to cry about, which I did every Friday night when I had the house to myself after mum went to her weekly bingo session. And it was during these nights that I constantly thought about the best way to end my life.

The pain didn't stop there. My brother, who was an alcoholic, had to move back home with mum and me, and this caused us a lot of pain. I watched as my brother

suffered from this horrible affliction and I tried so hard
to help him. But he too must have been suffering
something deep inside to make him drink so much.
The last straw was when I found him in so much agony
that I called an ambulance to rush him to hospital, where
I sat with him for hours. He was told that if he drank
again, he would die. And that's what he needed to hear to
finally make him stop.

At 15, I started working, and earning money felt really
great. But all I really thought about was helping my mum
and family and trying to get myself the things I needed
and to keep up with what my friends had. I didn't know
then that spending would soon become an obsession for
me.

Spending was something that made me feel so great, but
eventually it would also help me get into over £50,000
worth of debt with very little to show for it. Not knowing
how I could best deal with this much debt, I got some
advice and after looking at all my options I decided to
enter into an Individual Voluntary Arrangement. This
meant I would have to live off very little money for five
years, but that I would be debt-free as a result. I have just
over a year left at the time of writing and wow, this has
been a challenge, but soon I will be free of debt.

As for relationships, well, I had many, and they all failed
because of the feelings I had towards men, and the low
self-esteem and low self-respect I had for myself. I
allowed myself to be used by men, and was also raped,
but never bothered doing anything about it because I had
just given up on anyone really caring.

One day I thought that I had found the love of my life,
but because of all my negative emotions, I had just

136

brought another liar and cheat into my life. I so wanted to have a baby with this man (why you wonder?) and to be like all my friends who were having babies. And I really thought that after all I had been through, I would be granted this one thing.

But, after four years of trying to conceive, an early miscarriage, and an operation to tell me that I had endometriosis, I found out that this man had cheated on me and got someone else pregnant. I felt like my world had ended.

Well, that's all the bad stuff.

Now for some good stuff...Yes there is good stuff and there will be much more to come ☺.

While I was experiencing all of this, I always felt something inside me saying 'Helen, you must keep going.'

After leaving school with one grade C, I decided to go back and try again. I completed a GNVQ while redoing some GCSEs and after this I did some 'A' levels. I then decided to go to university and completed an Art & Design course and a degree in Graphic Design. I did all this whilst working part-time to support myself and my mum with bills.

After university I didn't know where I was going as I lacked confidence in my abilities. I got a job in a bank and worked my way up to become a manager. After being made redundant from this role, I tried other jobs, but never really felt I fitted in. I finally found a job I loved after being made redundant for the second time. This involved managing a centre where we supported people back into employment.

137

I loved this job as I felt I could use my many experiences to try to help others.

I've always worked hard but felt that I lacked confidence and had low self-esteem. My friend Lisa helped me to see that there were people out there who really wanted to help me and make me believe that I could feel different about myself. I decided to start going to church, where I found a lot of peace.

It was at this point I decided to come out to my family about all the pain I was suffering inside. It was a very hard time for us but my family were there for me and supported me fully. I love them dearly and don't blame them for anything. I then chose to be baptised and chose to forgive the person that abused me.

Forgiving them meant that I could finally move on with my life and get rid of all the anger inside of me. I felt that being baptised really helped cleanse my soul. It is from this point that I chose to change my path, to begin a new journey.

Over the last few years I have been on a journey of rediscovering ME. I say ME in big bold letters because that's who is most important to me now.

I had dealt with all the bad stuff in my mind by disposing of it, and now I needed to start filling my mind with good stuff. I would write down every positive or motivational quote I saw in a little book and carry this around with me and keep referring to it.

Next, I started reading. Reading a lot of self-development books, and books about how other people had changed their lives. I met some wonderful people, and joined a supportive mastermind group. Next I took an NLP Practitioner course and worked towards gaining coaching and counselling qualifications. I also started voluntary work to help other survivors of abuse.

My aim is to start my own business helping others see that they can also choose to change and create a new life for themselves, a life without pain, fear or hurt or feeling that they are not good enough. And create a new life where they always feel happy but, most of all, fall completely in love with themselves and all that they are.

EXERCISES:

1. Write
Writing is such a powerful tool. Everyday write down your personal feelings and thoughts, let it all out. If there is no one around to talk to, then this is a good way to clear your mind of what's going on in there and help deal with issues that you don't know how to handle. As long as you can get all these thoughts and feelings out of your mind in some way, you are helping to cleanse your mind and making it ready for new information to go in.

If you feel that a person has hurt you in some way or you don't agree with something they have done, then write them a letter about how you feel and then seal the letter and destroy it. That way you have expressed how you feel without making them aware of it and it is then dealt with.

This will help you move on.

2. Have a gratitude jar
Get an old jar and some pieces of paper and everyday write down something that you are grateful for or something great that you have achieved that day and put

the piece of paper in the jar. This will help you focus on the good stuff and not the bad stuff and the more you focus on the good stuff you will start to shift what your mind focuses on. And at the end of the year look back on all the things that you were grateful for to fill your heart with joy and your mind with happy and positive thoughts.

3. Change your physiology

This is really simple and can help change the way you feel in a second. Sit up straight and smile, and as soon as you do this you will begin to change your feelings. Or you could try dancing around your home or going for a walk, but always with a smile on your face. Getting up and being active is one of the most important things in life. It gives you energy and keeps you healthy, not only your body but also your mind, and especially if you listen to inspiring music or motivational people at the same time.

Helen Killeen – since this book was first published so many amazing things started to happen in Helen's life. She met her wonderful husband Ian and now has two beautiful children. She is training to become a Counsellor to support others.

If you would like to learn more about Helen's story or have experienced similar situations, please contact Helen at helenckilleen@hotmail.com

RECLAIMING ME
Sue Williams

This is me, it's who I am, sick and tired
Of feeling a sham. I claim my courage, face
My fear, break through constriction of society;
Self-imposed limits, those initiated by parents, dear.

It's taken so long for me to find out, conquer
Interminable worry, dread and doubt.
Gain a sense of my genuine feelings,
Not bound by expectations sending me reeling.

I've carried a heavy burden incredibly long,
A yearning to impress, fit in, belong.
Yet, how can I be truly accepted,
When my sense of self is not at all strong?

I've taken time out to search and explore,
Investigate habitual refrain of "poor, unloved
Little me". Playing the victim kept me safe,
Conditioned by restrained reality.

Now I recognise the power of my own thought,
Sub-conscious nature I was never taught. Express
Myself authentically, not how "I ought". Honesty,
Truth, authenticity, sometimes struggle; often fly free.

One thing I know for sure, the more I continue
To embrace my feelings, create a life I adore,
Continuously claim the inner me, I truly experience
How magical living a multifaceted life can be!

MY OWN BOSS
~ *Becky Lee*

"Despite external appearances, it is our very own perspective on how
we view the world and its circumstances that makes it true for us."
Becky Lee

Monday 13 February 2012 felt like a very significant day
in my life – as if it would be the very last day that I would
ever be in full-time employment, working for a "boss".

Now this may not seem such a big deal to some people
but since I began sharing my story I know that it has
inspired a lot of others too, so I hope that it will help you
to understand why it was such a poignant day and also to
reach out to you in some way, however small that may be.

You see, ever since I was a teenager, I have always wanted
to be "my own boss" – to me this signified having total
freedom to call my own shots, to be a savvy business-
woman and, moreover, to be fully in control of my own
life, without ever having to answer to anyone else again.

Now you may be wondering, where did this over-
powering drive and need for freedom and independence
come from? This would be a good time for me to take
you back to my childhood, which was extremely
unconventional and extraordinary.

Everyone who has heard my story has been shocked and
listened in disbelief. The most common response after

the disbelief is that people are absolutely astounded to find what a calm and grounded person I am despite all that I went through. I have learnt that your "perspective" and how you deal with any circumstances that life throws at you will determine how successful and happy you are in life. So, I hope that this will help you to understand why freedom is so important to me.

Although I was born in Hampshire in England, I did not get to experience life in the UK until I was eight years old. My parents originate from Hong Kong and I was taken back there as a small baby, where my sister was born some 15 months later. Immediately after this my parents left myself and my sister in Hong Kong to be brought up by my grandparents, whilst they returned to the UK to begin their catering business. As a sad consequence of this I did not get to meet my parents again until I was eight years old and my sister was seven.

Coming to the UK was a huge shock for both of us and we were absolutely terrified – travelling to a new country thousands of miles away where we did not speak the language, encountering a new culture and effectively two "strangers" who were apparently called our "mum" and "dad". It was all completely new to us and we soon discovered that we also had another sister and brother who had been born in the UK after us.

Up until that point in my life, my grandfather had been the person I knew as my "parent" and caretaker and I missed him desperately and wished I could just be back home with him, where everyone and everything was familiar. I cried myself to sleep every night for years. From then on, things did not get any easier.

The worst thing was that my sister and I never formed that "bond" with my parents. They continued to work extremely hard and long hours on their business, trying to support their ever-growing family and leaving virtually no time to spend with any of us.

As a result, there was very little love and affection growing up in our household and, for those who have studied psychology, you will know that from the ages of one to seven is when a child develops all their beliefs and values, according to the world around them. So now I completely understand why I share so many similar values, traits and beliefs with my grandfather (and not my parents), despite not ever living with him again after I left Hong Kong.

During this time and throughout our teens, it was extremely hard for my sister and me to adjust to our new lives with this ready-made family of "strangers" we had been thrown together with. I became an increasingly frustrated person, displaying prolonged bouts of anger whilst my sister withdrew more and more into herself. My parents were also very strict and controlling. They gave us no freedom, so that aside from school, we had no interactions with others our own age, any other adults or family members.

And so, the feeling started to grow stronger and stronger every day that I would never follow in the same path as my parents. I would do whatever it took to become financially independent so that I would not have to go through what my parents had to with us. They completely missed out on our childhoods and I was determined never to let that happen to me and the children I would one day have.

I want to be there for them at every stage of their growing up, to be able to help develop and nurture them with love (the way that my parents never did), but most of all to have the precious time to spend with them – time that we shall never be able to get back again.

The one quality that I did learn from my parents was their extremely strong work ethic – although it may seem wrong to some, I had started to work in my parents' catering business since the age of nine.

During most of my teens, as well as attending secondary school, my sister and I worked every Friday, Saturday and Sunday night in the kitchen of my parents' business, as these were the busiest periods. And from the age of 16, I also took on a waitressing job all day Saturday and all-day Sunday, as well as school holidays on top of this schedule.

So, I spent all my time either going to school or working – which beat just being stuck indoors and not being able to go out. Trust me; working was definitely the better option back then!

This strong work ethic that I developed in my teens actually served me extremely well, leading me to excel in every job that I took on. You see, I had learnt that "working hard" was the only way to success and for many years thereafter this is what I did, keeping my head down and just getting on with the task in hand.

After gaining a Bachelor's (Honours) Degree in Law at university, I decided to turn down the offer of finishing my law finals at the prestigious School of Law in Guildford, Surrey. Instead I decided to get a job as soon as possible so that I could start earning money, which would then enable me to move out and support myself at the earliest opportunity.

I went on to build up an extremely successful career in sales for myself, taking on roles within the retail, holiday, car and property industries, where I regularly achieved sales targets. I also won multiple accolades and prizes in every single one of my posts, such as "Top Performer of the Year" and "Best Office/ Branch" etc.

You see, my "belief" in creating my own freedom for myself was very strong. I thought that the only way to achieve it was to create a sound financial life that allowed me to look after myself and not have to rely on anyone else ever again.

After my horrendous childhood experience, it was this "belief" that drove me to extreme success and recognition in every single role that I took on. But don't get me wrong, I actually thoroughly enjoyed all my roles. Not only did I gain regular promotions and financial success, but I also got to meet some fantastic people and travel to some lovely places.

The ironic thing was that the "love" of taking on a new role and challenge was always far more important to me in every single case than the lure of the money – not that I knew it at the time but it is so true that "if you truly love what you do then the money follows". So, one of the big lessons that I have learnt is to follow your heart and do what you love.

I also had the fantastic opportunity to move to and work in Spain for a year, near Barcelona. This was one of the best decisions I have made as it completely opened my perspective and broadened my experience of life. After having an inner yearning for years – I just loved anything and everything about Spain – I followed my heart.

During this time, I not only purchased my own home but I also started to purchase other investment properties, so beginning my journey into the property world. After making some money from my very first property as an investment rather than my own home (which happened quite by accident but that is another story!) I had a massive light-bulb moment. This stroke of luck made me realise that property was a possible answer to earning myself the freedom that I was so desperately seeking. I became extremely excited.

The other great thing was that it meant I would still have the security of my day job whilst I developed more properties (as you can imagine, security was such a precious value of mine after my insecure childhood). Despite the lack of any kind of love or happiness in my childhood, I have since come to accept that I would not be the person that I am today had it not been for my unconventional upbringing.

I am now truly grateful as it has helped to turn me into the person that I am today – a positive, compassionate, resilient and financially savvy independent woman who has created an abundantly contented life for herself. My adversity had actually propelled me with the drive and "belief" that I could achieve whatever I wanted in life. This feeling was so strong in me and I was so single minded about it that there was no other possible outcome – no other options even entered my mind.

Slowly but surely, I started to gain just that little bit more freedom in my life. Now the freedom is not just based on financial independence but also the time and space I need to find peace and acceptance of myself. Leaving my full-time employment was one of the very last freedoms that I needed to achieve personally; hence I hope you can understand a little bit more as to why this was such an important milestone for me. If we look hard enough, we will always find positives to be learnt from all the adversities that we face in life.

EXERCISES:

It has been widely documented and researched that one of the best things that we can do is to practice gratitude in our lives on a regular basis. Not only will this make us see and appreciate just how much we already have in our own lives, but it will also help us to search for and find all the positive things, people and circumstances which we will continue to be grateful for.

This is a great way to train our mind to automatically see the best of every situation, circumstance or thing rather than focus on the negatives immediately. Done over time, you will see dramatic results in your outlook on life, which in turn will also lead you to notice the improvements in all areas of your life.

I like to do this simple exercise just before I go to bed so that I drift into sleep at my most optimum and positive state, being so grateful for everything that has happened in my day. This also helps positivity to seep into my "unconscious" mind, which research has shown is so many times more powerful than our "conscious" mind.

Before you baulk at having to come up with five good things that happened to you each day (which a lot of my clients initially do when I ask them to try this exercise!) – I must reassure you that it really is not as daunting as it sounds! Once you get into the swing of it, it gets easier and you will be surprised that you may actually start to enjoy it and look forward to completing it every day!

149

To create this daily ritual, follow the steps below:

1. Purchase a notebook or journal.

2. Every night, just before you go to bed, write the date
    at the top of the page and list five things that you are
    grateful for which happened to you or that you
    experienced that particular day – these can be
    anything from major to minor, e.g. getting that job
    offer to the sun was out, moving into your new home
    to a smile from a stranger in the street, getting a new
    client to having a roof over your head, etc. It does
    not matter what it is, the most important thing is
    what made YOU feel grateful on that particular day,
    and this can vary from day to day.

3. Try this consistently for two weeks and notice any
    changes in your outlook and attitude towards your
    life.

4. Ideally, continue this as a part of your daily routine.
    The results will just keep on improving for yourself
    and all those around you. If you can, increase the
    number of things that you are grateful for to ten.

Becky Lee is a property investor with properties both in
the UK and abroad.

This Whole New Chapter is All About Me
Sarah Klugman

I step out into an open space
No longer participating in the chase
I'm not the type to run or flee
This whole new chapter is all about me

Fear, I've let go of his hand
Strong and proud is how I stand
My mind and soul are flying free
This whole new chapter is all about me

In stillness I think I hear your heart beat
I see your face when I walk down the street
My heart it quickens, it fills will glee
This whole new chapter is all about me

So, I walk alone, filling up with life
And slowly, I am removing the knife
Life is uncertain and that's how it should be
This whole new chapter is all about me

Time has become my new best friend
With each passing day my heart will mend
My spirit is ripe; it's fallen from the tree
This whole new chapter is all about me

LESSONS FROM ADVERSITY
~ *Dr Claire Maguire*

"Life has no smooth road for any of us; and in the bracing atmosphere of a high aim the very roughness stimulates the climber to steadier step till the legend, over steep ways to the stars, fulfils itself." W.C. Doane

Several years ago, I wrote out my dream: to open a retreat centre. I put it to one side, not knowing how I was going to make it a reality. For if I looked at the facts – the hows, the scale of the dream, what was involved – well, I had to admit I had no qualifications to do such a project. I had no experience; I didn't even know what exactly happened on a retreat.

Yet something in me was pulled to the idea of running a place where women could come together and explore areas of their lives in a safe and nurturing environment. As I visualised it, felt it in my body and heard the laughter as women shared their stories, I planted the seed of belief that I could do it in my mind.

I started the steps to fulfil my dream: learning, training, connecting. And yet, my plans took a serious diversion, in the form of adversity, as I was diagnosed with breast cancer. Needless to say, I was devastated, shocked and in disbelief – for how could this happen to me?

I was only 37, I was forging ahead making great progress with my coaching business, I was in the best physical

152

shape I had ever been and I was excited about life. It all appeared so unfair. And it meant I had to energetically step away from my business, my passion for working with women and my flair for using raw food as a tool for transformation.

The cancer treatments left no space for me to deal with others. It left me to retreat into myself, allowing for discovery through deep self-exploration, spiritual connection and exquisite self-care. I became my top priority and I learnt many lessons about life.

Throughout this period, I always held onto the belief that I would survive, that I would get through it and go back to my coaching business. This unwavering belief kept me focussed, motivated and inspired.

As I entered back into my life, back to business, back to the everyday world, I felt pure joy that I was alive and well. But there was something inside me that felt unsettled, for I had experienced profound shifts in my perception of life. I had dealt with so much emotional pain, that I was in effect a new person. However, I wasn't expressing this new me through my work. Instead I was trying too hard to be what I used to be, thinking that was somehow better than who I had become.

I had stepped back into the business role I had created before breast cancer, entitled The Raw Bombshell; she was all about being hot, sexy and raw. She was all about the body, and was incredibly noticeable with her bright red hair and slinky body. Obviously, with chemotherapy I had lost my trademark hair, gained weight and was now not all about raw food. And yet I was still trying to be The Raw Bombshell as if this was the best version of me. It hurt.

I knew more, had learnt more, and had so much more experience and wealth to offer the world. Trying to be someone I wasn't created a massive feeling of disharmony and an incongruent approach to my teaching.

This feeling was heightened after a massive operation of reconstructive breast surgery. This operation was physically hard as my body struggled to overcome the mutilation, and emotionally scarring as I came to terms with the lasting effect of cancer.

As I sought to deal with these effects and to move forward, the opportunity finally arose to make my dream of running a retreat centre a reality. With the family home nearing completion of an extensive restoration project and my step-mother looking for a business to run from it, we spoke at length about my dream to run retreats. It seemed like the perfect win-win situation.

The bringing myself into the present moment, the letting go of the emotional pain, the self-care I gave myself and being true to who I was now, enabled me to fully embrace my belief that yes, I could contribute my gifts to the world; that yes I could congruently and authentically share my stories and teach my lessons learnt.

154

I had learnt to effectively let go of stress, to master my emotions, to stop judging myself against others and to say goodbye to the comparison game of me not being good enough. I learnt to deal with the negative chatter, and to accept myself whatever was going on. I had to step up and get out of my own way, to go for it. I had to really believe in my gifts and to see that I was there to act as a vessel for other women's transformation. It wasn't all about me!

Within a short seven months after the surgery I had opened the retreat at Split Farthing Hall in Thirsk, North Yorkshire, and had stepped up to lead my very first retreat. In front of me were wonderful women who allowed me to facilitate their exploration of self-discovery. It was amazing. I heard the laughter that I had previously envisioned. I was humbled, grateful and inspired.

In just over a year, I had the privilege of leading 23 retreats. Throughout all that time I held onto my strong belief that yes, I can achieve my dream. The belief in my abilities allowed me to effortlessly create five different themed retreats. To believe that yes, I could deliver an experience enabled me to deliver deep and meaningful results. To believe that I could facilitate transformation and inspiration made it possible for me to put myself in a role I had never had before.

It was all a leap of faith, a big giant leap. And the feedback has been more than I could have ever dared imagine. To witness the smiles on my guests' faces is priceless. To know that I never faulted on my belief, that I never shied away from my gift, that I never hid my shining light and in doing so I turned my dream into a reality – that is just fabulous.

How can my story help you in your belief? Firstly, I would love you to know that when you ground yourself completely in your dream, when you are unwavering in your passion, it allows others to reflect belief back to you, which heightens your belief. This process enables you to invite people to share your vision. This in turn creates the momentum for you to turn your dream into a reality; for I have found it takes more than you alone.

How then can you create this strong belief? From the lessons I learnt in overcoming my personal adversity I would like to share with you the following:

Be in the present moment. Allow the past to be the past and don't worry about the future. Don't take the "what ifs" and "if onlys" with you and don't let the stress and the worry of how to do it take over. By being in the present you become centred and allow emotional pain to dissolve.

The most effective way to do this is to breathe deeply and consciously; be aware with all your senses of what is around you. To understand that at that moment nothing is out to get you and that you are not in harm's way. To trust that everything will be OK and life will unfold, in mysterious ways, according to your deepest desires.

Be kind to yourself. Create an exquisite self-care ritual, one that nurtures and nourishes you on all levels: physically, emotionally and spiritually. Do one thing that you are passionate about every day. Plus make sure that every day you nurture yourself with devotion, eat food that loves you and partake in movement that adores you. Make time for yourself, for you are the most important person. As you start to love yourself, your respect for who you are increases and this intensifies your belief that yes, your gift, your shining light, is worth sharing with the world.

Be true to who you are. Don't try and be somebody else. Don't try and be who you used to be. Identify what makes you, you. What are your qualities, what are your attributes, what do you believe in, what makes you tick? As you get really clear about what makes you special, the fear of making a bold move dissipates and you find it easier to identify and connect with like-minded souls. With people that are keen to hear your message and eager to communicate meaningfully with your gift. Enjoy the process and don't cling onto "right" ways and "wrong" ways. Just be you.

Dr Claire Maguire, a well-being and food coach, is the creative programme director at The Retreat at Split Farthing Hall, a place where women come to be inspired to take the next step towards living a fabulous life. For more information see www.splitfarthinghall.co.uk

I BARE ALL
~ Elaine Clark

I used to think I had no worth,
an insignificant speck upon the earth.
You see, I had no self-belief
could not accept what lay beneath.
Out to the world I would not look,
did hide myself inside a book.

Then a dream evolved within my heart
to delve into the world of art.
It was certainly never my intention
to outrage; nor flaunt convention,
Just a creative urge that I'd aspire
to simply discard all my attire!

Standing still. Limbs softly aching
Strange sensations I'm embracing.
I'm here before you! Standing tall
So proud that I am baring all,
in my birthday suit, as nature intended.
Just being me! Nothing amended.

Empowered! Self-love I did achieve.
Now in myself I do BELIEVE.

REWRITING THE RULES
FOR THE NEXT GENERATION
~ Allison and Abbi-Louise Marlowe

"There's the right way, wrong way and YOUR way." Michael
Neil

Ecuador June 2012

Something truly magical happened that day – driving back
to our hacienda after horse riding western style across the
most magnificent and tranquil setting of Zuleta;
something deep stirred inside.

Why on earth was I denying my 15-year-old daughter the
opportunity to spend two weeks with me as part of her
school "work experience"? In a moment of rashness, I
sent her a text message, not even considering the time
difference between South America and the UK.

"Would you still like to do your work experience with
me?"

Almost instantly, despite thousands of miles apart, my
phone bleeped and I read the response "YES PLEASE".
It was one of those life-defining moments.

Back in the UK, Abbi and I talked about how this could
work.

"...here's one condition though Abbi – if you spend your work experience with me, you need to create your own project to manage."

As someone keen on amateur dramatics, Abbi had spent weeks contacting local theatres, hoping for an opportunity to spend two weeks behind the scenes and learning about life in the theatre. Nothing, it seemed, was working out and with all roads leading to an apparent dead end she was forced to look for an alternative placement, and found a local bistro willing to take her on.

I knew she was disappointed, yet at the same time I was reluctant to encourage her to watch over my shoulder. Wasn't that just taking the easy way out? After all, how much "experience" can working from home offer a youngster about the world of work in a "real life" setting?

Yet during that bumpy drive back to our hacienda, my intuition nudged me into action. I had no idea where this would take us. However, deep down it felt intrinsically the right thing to do.

Little did I realise it at the time, but Abbi already knew precisely what she wanted to accomplish…

Abbi-Louise:
When I was 14, I travelled to the Friends of Mulanje Orphans (FOMO) orphanages in Malawi. I was one of eight pupils selected to go on this trip. In order to go, I had to raise £1,500. No hand-outs from parents – this

160

was something we had to fund by ourselves and it was hard work!

It took me almost 12 months of car washing, jumble sales, cake baking and numerous sponsored events to reach my target.

Visiting Malawi was the most amazing experience of my life. When we arrived, I was totally overwhelmed by the welcome and feelings of joy. So much so, that my eyes filled with happy tears. During our stay we visited nine of the 13 FOMO centres where the orphans would come each day to be together and receive their one daily meal of rice and beans. It shocked me to see how happy these children were considering how little they seemingly had.

FOMO had grown from small beginnings in 2000 to care for over 5,000 children via a network of 13 centres covering over 85 villages in the Mulanje district of Malawi.

During our visits we played games, sang and danced with the orphans and presented the young children with clothes, school and sports equipment we'd brought with us as an offering. Everyone was grateful for the material things we gave, but the most important thing was just being together.

There was a real exchange – I taught the children how to play a variety of English games, such as "What's the time Mr Wolf" and "Hot Potato". In return I learnt how to be

161

really happy in the moment, something that we are not so great at doing in our country. I stowed so many wonderful memories and made friends for life; I knew I had to go back.

When that text message came through from mum, my heart skipped a beat. I wanted to use the two weeks to create a fund-raising project to fulfil my dream of returning to Malawi.

With the help of a web designer and a few others, I created an online venture, offering business-building products in return for a monetary donation.

Mum invests in her personal and business development and works with some of the leading female entrepreneurs in the world. She encouraged me to reach out and asked them to donate a downloadable MP3 recording or video product, something that was designed to help other women become successful faster in their business than if they were going at it alone.

At first, I wasn't that confident because I'd never done anything like it before but, having the support of someone who had run a similar project, along with my strong passion, it was a huge success. I managed to raise more than $2,500 in just over a week! (SO much faster than before!)

So, in July 2013, I went back to Malawi, creating even more wonderful memories a second time over. I would never have been able to raise a sufficient amount in such little time if I hadn't broken out of the mould and tried something different.

I'm not saying it was easy. It took lots of effort, at times I wasn't confident and co-ordinating a project this size was completely new to me. But if I hadn't believed in myself, I would never have got there. I learned not to be afraid to ask for help; the worst that could happen was that people would say no. This did happen; you just move on to the next person and keep persevering.

I now know I am able to repeat this process and raise funds online again, but more importantly I know that if I have faith in myself, I can do absolutely anything!

Allison Marlowe:
When we allow ourselves to be quiet and listen to our hearts, we usually know exactly what we need to do.

Society has imposed values and standards upon us and much of the time we go along with them, without even giving them a second thought. Society's rules and beliefs, for example the stories about money we have picked up and continue to feed ourselves, have become so ingrained in our conscious and subconscious minds that we barely recognise them as not belonging to us.

As we returned from Zuleta along the bumpy dirt track, it felt like time was standing still, there was a calling to follow my heart.

163

All too easily I could have packed Abbi off to the bistro, but I would have had to live with the notion that it would have had little impact on her self-esteem and personal development.

Our younger generation need to have a strong sense of self-belief instilled in to them and to not be afraid of their power, to embrace their creativity and believe in their dreams.

Children love to know they are of value to other people and can deal with situations occurring in their lives. It's essential to their self-esteem and cultivates qualities like responsibility, accountability and leadership. Yet this won't happen unless we provide a role model by being the best version of ourselves.

Sadly, our current society, and in particular our education system, is doing little to support this development. Creativity has been quashed, children are being taught to pass exams, rather than to learn. They are being taught how to conform rather than think for themselves.

What kind of futures are we paving for them? Self-belief is the foundation of our consciousness, determining everything about our lives. It determines the degree to which we feel, think and believe ourselves to be worthy.

I believe that it is time for more of us to wake up and to be who we are truly meant to be in this lifetime. Our cultural conditioning is no longer serving us or the world.

164

It's time for women in particular to reclaim their power –
to impact our families, our communities and even the
world.

Yet this won't happen if we continue to bow down to
cultural conditioning.

My own beliefs were challenged that day. It was time to
break the mould, rewrite the rules, to create a new way of
"being" that supported my truth.

Where had I picked up this nonsensical notion that Abbi
"should" go out and experience a "real life" work setting?
That didn't matter so much as how I was going to move
forward from this point on.

Marianne Williamson's most famous of quotes says "And
as we let our own light shine, we unconsciously give other
people permission to do the same. As we are liberated
from our own fear, our presence automatically liberates
others."

It was time to shine my light in order for Abbi to shine
hers. That was my purpose. It didn't once cross my mind
at the time how far the ripple effect of this initiative
would extend or the global reach Abbi would create.
I was told that Ecuador was a place where you will fall
back in love with life on earth and uncover the mysteries
of your life.

Little did I know the truth of that.

EXERCISES:

The following inspirational passage by Marianne Williamson is a favourite of mine ever since I first heard it. Take a moment and think about it. How are your beliefs impacting your life? For me, I know that my purpose is to be a great role model to my children. I don't always get it right but I do live with the purpose, knowing and intent that the next generation, our future, will lead fulfilling lives knowing "how" to think and create for themselves.

"Our deepest fear is not that we are inadequate. Our deepest fear is that we are powerful beyond measure. It is our light, not our darkness that most frightens us.

We ask ourselves: "Who am I to be brilliant, gorgeous, talented, and fabulous?" Actually, who are you not to be? You are a child of God. Your playing small does not serve the world. There is nothing enlightened about shrinking so that other people won't feel insecure around you.

We are all meant to shine, as children do. We were born to make manifest the glory of God that is within us. It's not just in some of us; it's in everyone.

And as we let our own light shine, we unconsciously give other people permission to do the same. As we are liberated from our own fear, our presence automatically liberates others."

Intuitive decisions

Many of us find ourselves being caught up in the frenzy of the fast-paced life of the 21st century. This is one of the exercises I share with my mentoring clients to help them make intuitive decisions:

Your intuition and imagination are very powerful tools worth developing.

If you need to make a decision, then imagine two alternative outcomes.

Step into the first option; imagine it in your mind. What can you see, feel, and hear, sense, believe?

Now project forward 10 minutes in time and check in again. What are you seeing, feeling, and hearing, sensing and believing now?

Now project forward 10 days? How do you feel now?

Now 10 years?

What is the consequence of making that decision?

If you are experiencing lightness, peace and joy then trust yourself.

If you feel fear, hesitation or contraction then this may not be the best decision for now!

Letting go to grow

The truth is the person you are today isn't the same person you were last year, or last month even! The past has served its purpose, yet if you find yourself clinging on tightly to old behaviours, attitudes and beliefs then you will continue heaving old energies along with you.

A lot of energy is used to keep our emotions suppressed, yet we often try to push them back down as if we are fearful of them, as if we might lose control if we were to release them. The thing is that emotions are not good or bad in themselves, and when we allow ourselves to feel them, get in touch with them, really feel them in the present moment; they will purely dissipate and disappear.

So next time you are aware of an emotion coming up for you, feel it and then choose to let it go. Examples of this could be a fear or anxiety of some sort, guilt, frustration, overwhelm, sadness, etc.

The best way I have found to demonstrate this letting go, is to ask you to pick up a pen or other small object that you would be willing to drop on the floor without giving it a second thought.

Pick something up right now and I will talk you through the process.

Hold your object, tightly in front of you and imagine it is one of those not so pleasant emotions, if you stood and held the object long enough it would start to feel uncomfortable. You may need to actually do this – if you do, be aware of the thoughts running through your mind. Now release your grip and roll the object in your hand, observe that you are simply holding this object and it is not attached to you!

The same is true for your feelings. Your feelings are not attached to you; we just hold onto them and "forget" we are holding on to them.

Now – let go of the object. Allow your hand to open and let it drop to the ground.

How difficult was that?

This is your opportunity to let go NOW; you can if you really want to. It is that simple.

Allison Marlowe, former founder of Global Winning Women, embarked on a new entrepreneurial project: The | Art | of | Pause. She is a firm believer that as role models for the next generation we are in danger of burning out. Allison teaches you how to move out of survival mode to maintaining a healthy long-term balance in your body's systems.
www.allisonmarlowe.com

Abbi-Louise Marlowe created The Science of Easy Fundraising aged 16, after accepting a unique opportunity to visit the FOMO centres in Malawi (Friends of Mulanje Orphans). Abbi-Louise has since become a mum. She is passionate about holistic living and plans to unschool her daughter.

The Entrepreneurial Revolution
Sue Williams

It's here, our decade, our yearned for solution,
Be bold, be decisive, it's called revolution!
No more the factory worker and the artisan,
Now, as entrepreneurial leaders, we plan
Our own futures; with our team we deliver
Outcomes and financial results that make you shiver
With excitement; yet for some trepidation,
Indictment of failure to act to achieve such elation.

Decidedly, a decade in which to be bold,
Through social media; mass communication takes hold!
Truly enough to "blow your mind"
As micro-niched on-line
"fruit label collecting" communities we find!
So, venture forth with passion into this electronic age,
Dominated by twitter, Facebook and LinkedIn business page.

Don't prevaricate, please make a pact,
Commit right now to urgently act!
Once applied, your business exploded,
At night to bed, you'll retire, financially loaded!
You'll have earned the right to swank,
On YouTube video, and will bank,
More cash from books, recordings and DVDs,
Bought avidly by fans, your loyal communities.
Built and nurtured through "know, like and trust"
Selling, you'll find, no longer needs thrust.
Rather, your clients, they'll flock to you,
Filled with rapture at all that you do.

I urge you, implement please, to truly earn success with ease!

171

MANIFESTING HEAVEN ON EARTH
~ *Mary McCallion Dempsey*

"Everything is possible for she who believes." Mark 9:23

When I thought about writing my story for this "Believe!" anthology, interestingly enough many came to mind. This was so good to realise and it reignited my belief in the power of belief once again. I hope it brings to mind your own magical stories.

As I was deciding which story I could do justice to, the one that seemed to ask to be written was about manifesting a house in my dream place – the place that I call "next stop heaven".

I first went to the Island of Achill, County Mayo, with my boyfriend and a group of friends. I fell in love with it immediately.

Along with a life-long romance with my boyfriend, now husband, began a life-long love-affair with the magical place of Achill. Probably cross-pollination! I would visit it as often as I could. It began to be my soul place – the one place in the world that seemed to sort me out and understand me. The women reading this will understand that it took a little bit longer for the other love to understand me!

I invite you to come with me in your wonderful imagination to this wild and beautiful island… allow your

172

mind to wander to the west coast of Ireland. You can easily cross to the Island of Achill by bridge... the island is surrounded by the wild Atlantic Ocean with beautiful majestic mountains of every shade and hue... purply browns, greeny greys, blues and orange pinks with red.

All are woven and blending into the mountains, creating a velvety backdrop to little white cottages, wandering pathways with stone walls decorating the wild and rambling landscape... you can almost smell the turf fires burning and taste the salt air. It feels protective; a safe caring atmosphere sprinkled all over it.

Your heart feels the rhythm and your soul resonates with the wild timeless earthiness. You feel the imprint of the divine everywhere, like you've found God's own painting canvas. Make yourself at home.

I always felt I belonged here somehow. So much so that I always dreamt quietly in my mind that I had a place to call home here.

When we got married and had our children, no matter what else happened we would always get ourselves to Achill for a few days. Sometimes we booked a house. This was usually a family home where the family moved in with granny for a few weeks in the summer season, and other times it was a caravan by the sea. No matter what it was – it was always a magical adventure.

One particular time stands out in my memory. It was 1989. We had booked a little house for a week. It was right beside the beach. It had great big rocks that you could jump across and lots of little rock pools. The weather was scorching. It was a kid's dream. They would get up in the mornings, togs on and straight down to the beach. The freedom they had on that holiday was priceless.

I remember my heart was so happy. We had been through an emotional roller-coaster and my life was in so such turmoil due to terrible family tragedies we had experienced…

This was just bliss. I remember sitting chatting with my husband and a few others one night, and we were enthralled by the beauty just outside the window. The moon shone and shimmered all over the water like it was treating us to a display. We were besotted. Someone said: "Look – angels dancing." Twinkly light skipped and danced on the water – it was so tranquil and childlike – it was magical.

I remember thinking "Imagine having this right outside your window." I sat mesmerised. It was like angels were physically connecting and communicating the joy that is possible. They were dancing and expressing the joy of heaven and I was totally in it.

We had three young children and were generally caught up in the daily run-of-the-mill things and getting by. But life had been an uphill struggle since my mother's death 11 years earlier.

You're probably curious as to why it would take so long to recover from my mother's death. Well, she was killed in a road accident and died at the young age of 47. She had 11 children and I was the oldest (23). I had just become a mother myself eight weeks earlier. You can imagine how hectic life had become as we all tried to deal with the intensity of her sudden loss. She was full of life, hale and hearty when she left the house that morning.

It was our first experience of death and the suddenness of that loss alone was horrendous to try to cope with. To see so many children having to face life without the natural comfort of their mother was heart-rending.

Sadly, eight years later, one of those children was to die suddenly too. He drowned while on holiday for the weekend with friends – he was 20. This broke our already hurting hearts even more. It seemed like we were in constant recovery and struggle with loss, trauma and grief. Family and friends were so kind and compassionate and it helped – but nothing could touch the depth of the sense of loss and suffering we were suddenly launched into.

Now, you can imagine the bliss of the night watching angels dancing on the water! That was one night that all was right with the world.

I was to remember this magical night. It is etched forever in my soul.

But now I'm going to ask you to jump 10 years into the future – now we are regular visitors to Achill. On one of those visits I wandered aimlessly from the house and down the rocks to the beach. On this particular day I felt a whisper!

"Look up." I looked up…

I said: "What?"

… "See… look again."

I saw it! My eyes welled up with tears of love and delight and I was rooted to the spot.

My Dream – I was looking at my dream now in reality, as if through the flashes of that memory of the angels dancing on the water.

You see, we eventually bought that house in Achill. I knew how blessed I was – and I call it "angel whispers" because I knew that the angels helped me manifest it against all the odds. But what I hadn't yet fully appreciated was just how much they had heard and how faithfully they fulfilled my wishes. Because, when I looked up, I saw that I was standing on the very same beach – the same rocks with the same view from my window that we saw that night 10 years earlier.

176

Not only did I get my house but I got my house in the exact spot that the angels and I had connected with heaven that night. These were the rocks my children had played on that wonderful summer holiday, creating an abundance of happy memories.

I was standing fully in my dream that once was in my imagination. It was as if I had walked into the picture that I knew so well. It felt like it was always meant to be and at the same time it felt like "How did this happen?"

I stood and knew how blessed I was (am) and how I had been listened to, and I felt so cared for.

For me, and now for my family it's the most spiritual place in the world.

Of course, it didn't just fall out of the sky, as my husband reminds me!

Looking back, here's how I see it unfolding:

THE BUILT-IN BLUEPRINT TO ACTIVATE:

1. Heart's desire – planting the seed in your heart (sow and nurture the seeds)

The blueprint comes from your deepest desire. Like anything on earth, everything begins as a thought, a word, an image, a dream. You can see it in your head – in your mind's eye – you can see the details, the colour, you can smell it, the scents that surround it, you can feel it, feel what it's like being there… as if you are there NOW.

2. Inwardly believing – I just knew this was going to happen.

I didn't understand how but "through heartfelt determination" you find the way.

Promise to myself and my family – create the way.
A lifestyle choice for now, that also ripples into future generations.

> "We are here to live mindfully in this life,
> We choose creativity, positive intent over unrewarding strife
> And as we choose to change how we ourselves perceive,
> in our own dreams, our legacy, our power,
> we truly believe!"
> (Sue Williams)

3. Intuitive actions – while going about my normal business I began to look at possible places – just for fun – even though I didn't have the way or the means to buy even a shed.

I returned to part-time work – second income for the first time. I got a better paid full-time job – doubled second income.

Guess what, I'm getting a whisper: "Let's be real here – the steps involved things like going to the bank and getting a mortgage. The house didn't just land out of the sky, but it also involved a new job to provide the means to pay for it in full with no stress or worries." Thank you, thank you – it's so good to remember that.

4. More angel whispers

Angels constantly whisper to each soul "There is no soul request too big."

"All that you desire already is – you couldn't desire it otherwise."

"What is for your highest good is for the highest good of all. This cancels out all thoughts of selfishness."

"When you ask and receive you receive for every person" – it's like you've filled your bucket more so you can give more."

And to finish here is one of my favourite pieces of scripture that runs through me constantly and I love having this opportunity to share it with you:

> "I came that you may have life and have it abundantly."
> (John 10:10)

God is on your side. Your dreams and desires are queued up, waiting for your request.

Pssst! You see, your beliefs are what put them on the conveyor belt for you to pick up.

What are you waiting for? You deserve the best life possible.

Write out your list – don't censor it, don't judge it, don't try to work out how. That's heaven's department. Yours is to attune to the desires already planted in your heart. Listen to them like you would listen to a dear child you love. Promise them. Believe in them. Allow them out to play and they will find their own way home.

Little note
Ten years later I took a training course with Doreen Virtue and I was taught the steps of manifestation.

I had been doing it without knowing that I was doing it. What a great surprise to look back and find this hidden in the steps of my own dream manifestation! I had followed my angel whispers not knowing that I was being guided in the natural laws and science of manifestation.

Mary McCallion Dempsey, founder of Angel Whispers, runs retreats that help people to develop into their true nature and calling. Mary also runs on-line workshops and one-to-one therapy sessions; and offers a quiet space for a solo writing retreat. See www.angelwhispers.ie

SHINE FOR ME
Sue Williams

As you remember me this day,
Let sweetness blend with sorrow,
You are my gift,
Left on this earth,
To create a brighter tomorrow.

And, as you ever blossom and grow,
My legacy lives on,
So be my light,
Within this world,
Through you, still brightly shone.

BREAKING THE RULES OF "REALITY" IS WHAT BELIEF IS ALL ABOUT
~ *Shuri Morgan-Radford*

"Growing up is losing some illusions, in order to acquire others." — Virginia Woolf.

Did you know that your life is just one big fabulous illusion?! Are you aware that it is an exciting movie in which you are the scriptwriter? Are you living your life as if every day is a "Holodeck"; an elaborate hologram that you are, in fact, creating? If not then "get with the programme" as they say! Your life will truly be remarkably different if you take this on – 100%.

This understanding is what I teach people and what I live by 24/7 and here's a fun story that illustrates just how the power of your belief is ALL there is – even when you are driving along a busy motorway!

I mentor a lady who lives in Alverstoke, which is about 14 miles from my home in Southsea. To get to her usually takes me about 40 minutes as it is a very busy road and there are almost always "snarl-ups" along the way.

However, on this particular day I'd had a visit from my father and step-mother and we (as usual!) hadn't stopped talking and laughing in enough time for me to eat my lunch and get myself ready.

As a consequence, I was only going to have 25 minutes to get to Allison! So, I decided to invoke all of the power of my belief in that journey, and here's how it went...

I set off and got on to the M27 to find myself speeding along in what my father would refer to as "boy racer" fashion. (Yes, unfortunately I revert to teenage-hood and change gender entirely when I get into my car!) I had started speeding because I had momentarily forgotten my belief that I would get there in time whatever the speed.

However, once I had reminded myself that I was creating the road ahead of me, I didn't have to wait long before a police car "appeared" in front of me. All of the cars had to slow down to a more sedate 70 mph! At this speed I could stay in the moment and just have a relaxing journey rather than consciously applying myself to the task, which made the journey so much more pleasant.

I exited the motorway and was trundling merrily along the start of the A32 when I had a brainwave inspired by a song! I had been hoping for some inspiration to explain something to my clients/students when there on the radio was the answer to my puzzle! The singer sang one word which sparked off a whole train of thought that gave me the answer! It wasn't convenient to stop the car so I let the thought go and decided to trust the fact that I would remember the idea later on.

Now, the direction that I take to Allison's has been set in stone long ago by my trusty sat-nav, whom I choose to call Gilbert. I didn't need Gilbert any more for this familiar journey, but could only follow his route without getting lost! Despite this, I reached one point on the A32 where it seemed like a great idea to take a completely unknown (to me) route marked Alverstoke! What fun!

I set off down a very long road that seemed to twist and turn this way and that and which apparently had no more markings for Alverstoke. Great! I was in the middle of nowhere, going nowhere. (Gosport isn't that big but it might as well be the moon when you've got my sense of direction. Yes – a faulty belief system which I need to change but you just can't do it ALL at once!).

Nevertheless, I was determined to keep my resolve to arrive on time utterly firm. I kept going down the road until I came to something that looked familiar – the sea! So, I decided to enjoy the ride and appreciate the sea; which I absolutely love, and to relish the fine, fresh October afternoon. However, due to the lousy-sense-of-direction belief I had to get trusty Gilbert out because I didn't know where Alverstoke had "disappeared" to.

So, I clicked on "Allison" but a further "problem" arose. Gilbert gets dead temperamental in Gosport! He has this "I-might-work-and-I-just-might-stay-asleep" kind of attitude! On this occasion he was in "sleep" mode. In spite of this, my resolve stayed firm yet again. Still determined not to be late, I decided to just pop round the next corner and see what would happen. Suddenly, Gilbert burst into life!

"In 50 metres turn left, then turn left and arrive at destination." Hurray! Allison's abode was in sight!

So, to recap – despite having had 15 minutes less to get to Allison's, plus having been "slowed down" by the police car, getting lost, plus the "sleeping" Gilbert, I parked up at Allison's with 4 minutes to spare; enough time for me to write down my radio idea, which incidentally, I used when mentoring Allison that afternoon!

You see, true belief doesn't just bend the rules of what we call "reality"; it can break them entirely. On this occasion it "suspended" time, something that has happened to me on many occasions.

As an aside, I once owned a 1972 Triumph Toledo called Merlin (we lived in Tintagel, North Cornwall, at the time so what else would you call your car?) which always got me everywhere on time despite its apparently ancient and dodgy mechanics! I may have a lousy-sense-of-direction belief but I also have a fab my-car-will-get-me-there-on-time belief!

Although I've given you a playful example of how it can work, belief is ALL we have. Life does not happen to us; it happens because of us. It doesn't happen from the outside in, it happens from the inside out.

As hard as it is to understand (and it can be even harder to actually practise constantly and consistently!) we write the script of our lives every day. Providing that your belief is strong and true, it can move mountains. There is only your movie/Holodeck/hologram and it's entirely up to you how you use it. Belief is your system for how you run your life whether in your relationships, your finances, your health or a simple car journey.

This awareness, along with "acceptance" its trusty bedfellow, has helped me through the most "difficult" of times. Acceptance should happen when things are going apparently "wrong". It's the reminder to ourselves that we have simply created the situation in order to move us to the next stage of where we need to be. Let me give you an example.

At the age of 22 I met a man who two years later became my husband. When I first met him, I found his personality to be interesting and he had that "dangerous" edge which made him exciting. I never quite knew where I was with him, but that just added to the knife's-edge feeling of being really alive. Every night that I arrived home my heart would beat hard not knowing what I would find when I walked in the door!

However, within a very short while, I began to realise that the "danger" that I was attracted to with this man was way out of control. The beating heart of excitement turned into abject fear as I began to understand the true nature of this person. He was actually a manipulating and controlling alcoholic who wanted to own me in every way and he saw it as his prerogative to make decisions on every step I took, whom I saw and how I spent my time.

186

It wasn't long before I was more than "dabbling" with alcoholism, illegal substance abuse and dubious sexual practices. I was also in deep depression, and his physical violence eventually put me in hospital with a broken jaw.

It took me a long and heart-aching eight years to fully realise that life with this man was never going to improve and that I would have to leave him even though I was actually still in love with him (believe it or not!)

I did leave him, and I gave myself some good recovery time in which I had to do some serious thinking about this whole experience. However, one thing was evident from the start. There was never any blame that I could attribute to my husband. "Why me" was never an option because on a deep mental level I had created this life for myself which included this violent man.

Although it was hard to accept, the outward experience was a reflection of my deeper feelings made manifest. I may not have had the "reality" that I had chosen directly but as Consciousness cannot tell you, it can only show you what you have going on in your mind and heart; it was showing me that there was a whole bunch of darkness that I was feeling towards myself.

It therefore followed that the only person to blame (although actually I don't believe that "blame" is a useful concept) was myself. The only person who could change that reality was me and not just by leaving him. I had to refrain from buying into the victim mentality or feeling sorry for myself because I had created this Holodeck all by myself! It then followed that once acceptance had kicked in, I could start to move forward in my life in the sure knowledge that I wouldn't have to repeat this scenario because I now understood (and more importantly, accepted) it.

The man I have been with now for 24 years (my second husband) is a kind, gentle, understanding, super-supportive and philosophical being who is about as far removed from my first husband as you could imagine! But of course, he is! I created him in my world of illusions, didn't I?!

THE TRUTH of how life actually works as opposed to how we are taught it works (since being knee-high to a grasshopper!), is how I live every single second of every single minute of every single day. I also love teaching others THE TRUTH through my work as The Consciousness Architect.

Sometimes I find it "easy" and I'm excited and blissful. Other days, when I forget what life is truly about, I fall momentarily back into "egoic victim". My life is full of games that I choose to play but many that I choose not to play; and so is yours. Your belief system is EVERYTHING. Whatever you believe will become your "reality" so be truly wise about choosing your beliefs!

Why not consider starting the process of reprogramming your Holodeck for happiness and contentment!

EXERCISES:

Here's how you too can begin to redesign your life:

1. Stillness meditation

Being still and in the moment is a great way to reconnect with Consciousness. It reminds you that life is actually about contentment, peace and love rather than what we are programmed to believe it is about, which is money, stress and suffering. So, take some time (preferable about 20 minutes) at the start of the day and then again around teatime to just sit with a lovely piece of music or simply in silence and remind yourself that Time doesn't actually exist. There is only NOW, this moment.

Make sure that you are sitting or lying somewhere comfortable and warm.

Take two slow, deep breaths in and out, allowing yourself to relax with each out breathe.

Let your breathing return to normal and concentrate on relaxing each part of your body starting with your feet.

When you have done this, tell yourself the following things. You don't need to use the exact words, just the essence is enough. Repeat the sentiment enough times to start to really feel the calm and stillness of being in the moment and letting everything else drift away:

"This is my time to relax.

I can allow myself these moments of peace to let any tensions drift away.

I give myself permission to let my mind relax.

I give myself permission to let my thoughts settle.

As thoughts enter my mind, I release them back into the ether. I let them go.

Right now, everything is exactly as it should be.

This is a perfect moment.

There is no past and no future.

There is only this moment. Now.

Thoughts may come into my mind but I can release them; I can let them go.

Right here and now I can be at peace.

Right here and now, my mind is still and calm and I recognise the value of silence.

Here, now, I can just be myself.

Here, now, I can simply be."

Don't berate yourself if you don't get it at first. Try again and really enjoy the time that you spend. There is no right or wrong way to do this; I have merely offered you a guideline. You may find your own way. Also, it is worth mentioning here that meditation isn't for everyone. Remember that in your Holodeck life there are no rules. What you choose to do is totally up to you!

2. The power of belief exercise
Next time you have an emotion you feel to be negative, un-resourceful or painful, take the following steps:

Ask yourself "Why am I choosing to do this to myself?"

Rather than suppressing the feeling, immerse yourself in it totally. Accept it.

Remind yourself that all of life is an illusion created by you; that your life is merely showing you what is happening in your heart and that you can take away the pain with the power of your belief.

Make a firm decision to remove the power from the moment.

Grasp hold of the emotion with your mind. (You may not logically understand what I mean by this but you will as you do it.)

Take a deep breath in and out, knowing that you are removing the power from the moment.

Resolve to always take responsibility for what you have created. Let the moment go and move on with your life.

This will not come easy at first. You will fight to remain a victim to the emotion. Don't give in. The more you practice the better your life will become – guaranteed!

Shuri Morgan-Radford is the author of *Authentically Yours Developing the Authentic Self.* She been a teacher and coach over for over 35 years. Her programme 'Harmonic Consciousness' teaches The Truth about the human experience through a blend of science, philosophy and spirituality.

FREE TO BE ME
Gill Potter

How do I feel about being me?
So many faces I show to this World
But no-one truly knows what it feels like to be me
I wish I could be open and free
Freed from this bondage of secrecy
So much stuff still in my closet
I need to look inside and clear it all out

So many lies and contradictions inherent within
And yet I'm the one so hung up on the truth
This double identity that I've lived with
Has given me the perfect cover for my purpose
But has also wreaked havoc in my life
To stand up and yell at the World
"Look at me – I'm so different and
I've fooled you all – everyone!"
Wow what a shocker – even to me!

It's taken 36 years to accept me
And I'm still scared of what lies within
It's so awesome and untouchable
But what is this undefined part?
That has driven me to the brink
of despair and insanity?
Only to transform at the 12th hour
to joy and enlightenment!
It must be God or the Divine spark
That I've tried to suppress and deny
Never believing I was good enough
Until now and I do believe I am enough!

So has everything else been a sideshow?
A form of escapism to prevent me facing up
to the real me and ultimate power
Of God versus my ego
So how does it feel to be me?

The constant unpredictable flux
Has been exhausting and at times exhilarating
Living on the edge of Divine madness
Masked by anything more acceptable
Addictions, obsessions, sickness
Anything was better than facing it!
The monster did eventually transform
And I guess the handsome Prince
will turn up some day and kiss me
And in that moment, I will know
In fact, that was when I did remember
But it's taken years to slay this dragon
And slay it once and for all
So that I might meet with YOU again

What is the magic elixir?

Love is the drug!
It opens every door
It takes you to the edge and lays you bare
It comes in many disguises
And weaves through the layers of your heart
Opening you up and intoxicating along the way
Until you're so drunk on ecstasy
You feel bliss-ed out of your mind
I remember – I am waking up!

And our Soul
Dances with joy
As it reaches its final destination
At long last – YOU are within reach!
Free the Spirit
And let it flow unbridled into my Soul
Every layer of my being overflowing
With Spiritual light until I am ablaze
This girl is on fire!

Lit up like a Christmas tree
Bedecked in tinsel and fairy lights
And able to relate to my World
And know it's ok to be me!
And by being me I am free!
And what is freedom?
It is God, love, enlightenment
Something worthy to die for!
Even the ego knows this!
And now that I've said "I do"
Knowing full well the consequences
I am free and I am freed
At long last
Permission to let go of my past!
Free to be me!

PICTURE THIS
~ Gill Potter

"I now release anything that is not for my highest good; any thoughts, any beliefs, any situations, any people, any forms or objects and I ask them to release themselves from me, and I let go easily, knowing that something better always comes for everything I release. I open to receive my higher good in every area of my life and I thank the Universe in advance for sending it to me – and so it is and so it shall be!"

Inspirational quote from my, Gill Potter's, journal at the time of the following events:

Picture the scene. It's a snowy January day and we have just entered a brand-new millennium with fireworks and parties all over the world. Everyone is excited about life; except me! Or so it seems…

Despite all of my hard work on my personal development journey to heal myself of Myalgic Encephalomyelitis (ME) something still feels very stuck!

My husband (Sandy) is looking for a new job as we want to move back to the Glasgow area, but nothing suitable is on the horizon. I'm reducing my anti-depressants as we also want to have a baby and start a new life together in 2000! I believe I can create the life of my dreams and be happy and well but my life doesn't seem to reflect it back to me (yet!)

196

I decide to listen to tapes by M. Scott Peck of "The Road Less Traveled" fame and as I do, something shifts. I pray and ask to align with my dreams and let go of previous old expectations.

Two days later I'm back in bed with a severe relapse from my ME (a chronic and debilitating condition which can last for weeks, months or years and has no known cause or cure in traditional medicine).

It's so bad I can't speak or think. When I open my mouth, nothing comes out. I'm terrified! My husband can't take care of me as he has to work 12-hour shifts; even making myself a cup of tea is beyond impossible when I'm in a relapse. (He later tells me that he's so angry with me for being ill again that he feels like killing me.)

My dad drives the hundred miles to our flat after my SOS call and virtually carries me out to his car, with my hurriedly packed suitcase and a couple of inspirational books and CDs.

By the middle of February, I am in despair. I can't sleep and I am in severe pain. My body feels worse than ever and I know it's probably related to reducing my anti-depressants. The neural pathways just don't seem to work anymore! I pray and surrender my life to God and divine will. Prompted by the Scott Peck tapes I ask to love God and myself first.

Sandy comes to visit me on his days off as I'm still at my parents' house trying to get well. By chance (or by divine design) he brings a complementary therapist magazine with him. It had arrived by post that same day. I vaguely remember I had ordered it before Christmas.

I open it up and the word SHEN jumps out at me. I see there is a therapist five miles from my parents' house and call her even though I can still barely speak.

She is lovely and has had ME too – so no need to explain to her how desperate I feel – she completely understands. She is one year younger than me and in remission from ME. I discover she has lost her partner in the last 12 months from cancer and is still in the midst of her own grief. I'm grateful for her understanding and willingness to visit me at my parents' home.

Within two days she has given me three sessions and something big is shifting.

Shen is an emotional release technique that helps the body to heal by remembering traumatic experiences that have been buried and may be deeply unconscious. Our mind may forget but the body never does. She skilfully releases the blockage and suddenly I am experiencing events from my past like watching an old black and white movie of stills, and hearing voices speak to me. I am back in Corfu in 1988 reliving a holiday romance with an Irish guy called Michael and new insights help me let go – at last!

I realise my holiday romance was probably just that and that it was God's will that it ended the way it did. I accept this, and I am more at peace with this new understanding. I let go at last!

I sleep well for the first time in one month. My arms start to be able to move above my head and my heart chakra is blown wide open.

I cry constantly for 24 to 48 hours.

Then I feel the greatest amount of love I have ever felt for myself and others. I am really healing this (ME) – at last! I am shown the deeper cause of the blockage and despite the fears, resolve it with the person who was related to the cause. The gift was to give me greater faith and I am able to forgive. Suddenly my life makes more sense, though it also opens up new levels of anger and vulnerability within me.

One month later and my body has returned to better health and I can start to do more normal things again. My husband has an interview for a job in Glasgow and everything is coming together.

I continue to receive weekly Shen and parts of my body that have felt dead and numb for years awaken. I feel immensely grateful to the Shen therapist and we become firm friends.

Life is still chaotic though, and my husband wants me to return to our home. I'm not so keen to move back to Dundee. It feels so isolating and I have unhappy memories of feeling trapped alone in our flat while he is at work. I agree on the condition that he WILL get a new job and we WILL move to the Glasgow area where I have more support from family.

So, four months after moving back to my parents' house I am able to go home with my husband. Our marriage, which had been on the brink of a break up, is still hanging by a thread.

I wake up on the first day after going home to the post. A magazine from LuminEssence in the USA looks of interest. I open it and see a course on "Transforming your Life with Divine Will". As I read it, an energy surges through my body, and I feel like I'm vibrating so much that I am thrown across the room.

It's May 2000 and beautiful outside. Much too beautiful to spend my life trapped in the past and to be ill forever! I order the taped course and one week later it arrives. I start listening to the journeys.

Within one week my husband has an interview for a job in Kilmarnock and is successful! I am jumping for joy! At last we can sell our flat and start a new life together! We put our two-bedroom flat on the market and hope for a quick sale.

Unfortunately, six other flats follow us on our street and it may not be so easy! The flat market in Dundee is depressed – just our luck! Still, I know everything happens for a reason, and I continue with my new course on manifesting my dream life.

I move back to my parents' and Sandy has to move to Kilmarnock and stay in a room at the nurses' home alone; we can't sell our flat and we can't afford to pay two lots of rent and our mortgage. Although my health has improved and I can do more than I have for years, I still can't work.

We search for solutions and I keep doing the spiritual growth course. By September I feel a bit disheartened and pray for guidance.

I am focusing on manifesting a new house for us and better health – a new start and a new life. I study astrology and can see I am on track, so I keep my faith!

Something shifts and a miracle occurs. Persimmon homes are offering part exchange. We go to see the houses (and I fall in love with them) – they are three-bedroom semi-detached houses with a driveway. They even have an en suite shower room, downstairs toilet and a big family bathroom. This exceeds my wildest dreams. There is a great dining kitchen with patio doors and the house has a wonderful view over the fields and is in a beautiful location.

We agree terms, and despite losing money on the part exchange deal (on our flat) we gain big time, and move into our brand-new house on 30 November 2000. My life and health have turned around and I am ready to really start anew! Ten months after feeling I may never recover from ME, I am now in much better health, my husband has a new job that he loves, I have supportive family and friends around me and everything has fallen into place so beautifully!

That is the power of believing in your dreams AND taking the guided actions to manifest them!

EXERCISES:

1: How to feel in the present and release negative emotions
Accept this is how you feel. Don't deny, resist your feelings, or distract yourself. Avoid turning the negative emotions into anger.

Say what you feel to the person who has caused the hurt (or write a letter to them or speak it out as if they are with you, if you no longer have any contact with them).

Let go and move on – be grateful for the opportunity to heal yourself and your life and to be free of the past.

2: Becoming love

Listen to one of the following suggested songs each day for a week. Sing the words to yourself (in the mirror) and remind yourself that love starts with you as you sing! Journal on your experiences after doing so and record how you feel before and after each song.

- You are beautiful - Christina Aguilera
- Flying without wings - Westlife
- You are so beautiful - Joe Cocker
- You don't know you're beautiful - One Direction
- Loving you - Minnie Riperton
- Love will save the day - Whitney Houston
- When love takes over - David Guetta ft. Kelly Rowland

Listen to these or your own favourite love song(s) that inspire you.

3: Truth telling

When you tell the truth, you plant new (healthy) seeds of love in your life, and divine grace works FOR you. Often when we lie (to self or others) we block the very grace and miracles we seek – so tell the truth to yourself first and then to others – ALWAYS!

Ask to be shown the truth about your life.

Pray or write this in your journal – show me the hidden things that block me from knowing the truth of my life, help me to live my mission with more success, ease, grace and joy.

Be open to new answers and record insights, thoughts, ideas and dreams after you have asked or prayed about the above.

Take the next step or action you feel will move your forward.

Trust and let go!

Gill Potter is a writer working in healing modalities to support clients by sharing proven methods of transforming into your best self. She is working on a new book project.

You can contact Gill at yoursacredpurpose@gmail.com

BELIEVE
Hannah Imogen Jones
Visionary poet, photographer and creative

Anything is possible
Attainable
Achievable.

There's just one rule -
The goal must be
Unto yourself
Believable.

LOOKING AT LIFE
THROUGH A NEW LENS
~ Sarah Presley

"We don't see things as they are, we see things as we are" ~ Anais
Nin

"Mum, I just don't see the point of life anymore".

I didn't want to end my life; I just could no longer see any
point to living. Mum didn't see it this way. She thought
she was going to lose me forever. I saw the fear in her
eyes, as she sharply sucked in a breath. And with that, the
strangest thing happened – I could feel myself floating
out of my body and floating into her body. There I was,
looking at me through her eyes. I could feel how she was
feeling. She felt desperate. She felt scared. She felt
hopeless.

With a blink of an eye, I was back in my own body. I
remember reassuring her, "I'm going to be ok; I'm going
to sort it out". I wanted to say anything to get her to
release the fear in her eyes. But her eyes were only
reflecting the fear she had seen in my eyes. And her
feelings were reflecting my own. I could tell she didn't
believe me. But something else had now set inside me. I
could feel determination. But more than that, I could feel
belief in myself that I could turn this around.

This happened in 1999. I was a shell of my former self
and feeling like all my inner lights had been switched off.

I had been completely derailed from everything I had known before. I felt exhausted, sad and scared. Depression and anxiety were a by-product of the symptoms, and some days the fatigue was so great it would even hurt to blink. I had been told it was highly likely I would feel this way for the rest of my life, and this was a bitter pill to swallow. I had completely lost the point of living, and although I wasn't suicidal, I couldn't find any joy in life. I was 26 and I had been diagnosed with Myalgic Encephalomyelitis – M.E.

Prior to M.E. I had lived life at one million miles an hour. From a young age, I had been a sponge to all the emotions I could feel around me. I never knew what to do with these emotions, so I just buried them and kept myself as busy as possible and tried not to think about them too much. I was in a rush to grow up. I bought a house at the age of 18, I was married by the time I was 21 and I was divorced by the time I was 23. At the time of diagnosis, I was living with my boyfriend.

I had been balancing my full-time job in an office alongside a UK tour where I was singing in a band that was supporting a well-known group. We were on the cusp of a music career, and we were being courted by the record industry. I was a people pleaser - I was working hard to keep the bosses in my office happy with my work and at the same time I was playing hard with my band. But trying to keep everyone happy was making me feel really anxious.

I also referred to myself as "the born worrier". In fact, if I didn't have anything to worry about, I would worry! It is no wonder my mind and body gave up on me. I had ignored and buried all the warning signs. Little did I know at this point, having M.E. was actually going to be the best thing to happen to me. It was going to give me the opportunity to be reborn, to start looking at life through a new lens and with a new and improved perspective. I was going to awaken, to heal, and to have a new appreciation for life.

After the conversation with my mum, I didn't have a clue where to start. My doctors recommended I looked at my diet, plus I started to see various complementary therapists and read every self-help book I could get my hands on. All of them were extremely helpful and all were so incredibly relevant to my healing journey. But it was a book on Buddhism that became life changing for me, although at first, I almost dismissed it.

I read a chapter about meditation amongst many other sections of the book. This talked about how we are a vibration and how everything in the universe has its own vibration. And if we repeat a mantra (i.e. a word) we can become the vibration of the mantra. The book suggested I repeat the word "Om" (believed to be the sound of the universe) but I really didn't want to "Om". I just couldn't relate to "Om". I couldn't see myself oooooooohoohhhhmmmm-ing!

So, I decided it wasn't for me. But as life continued, I couldn't get the thought of meditation out of my head and the idea of becoming a different vibration. I thought about what words I would like to "be". I decided I wanted to be "happy, healthy and strong". So, I followed the instructions in the book and picked one of these words at a time as a focus. Sometimes I found it easy to meditate and sometimes it was hard. But I was really hooked. In fact, I did it as much as I could.

I would do sitting meditations. I would do meditations when brushing my teeth or washing the dishes. Over time, I started to see a difference with my health and wellbeing. My sleep patterns began to improve and I would feel more rested from sleep. My mind became less foggy and more focused. I also began to feel a bit more resilient too. But I still felt like my lights were switched off.

Luckily for me, reiki was going to change this. After receiving the attunements to reiki in 2003 I connected even deeper into the understanding of the vibration of my own personal energy. I could see the impact my negative thoughts and emotions were having on my mind and body. And with the beautiful healing energy of reiki I could feel my lights were switched back on.

On a daily basis, I would use the various techniques I had learned through meditation and reiki to worry less, and I began to focus on what was right in my life instead of focusing on what was wrong. I was less harsh on myself and started to treat myself kindly. By the end of 2003, I had shaken the shackles of M.E. and I really had become "happy, healthy and strong". The belief in myself had paid off.

Having learned so many tools to bring me to a place of living a healthy and well-balanced life, I decided to help others who were going through a tricky time in their lives. After extensive training I set up my own Holistic Therapy business, supporting people to find a natural balance to their mind, body and spirit.

I also embarked on a Reiki Master apprenticeship, as well as a City and Guilds Level 4 certificate in Further Education Teaching. Since 2011 it has given me the greatest pleasure to help empower individuals in the various levels of reiki, as a Reiki Master Teacher.

In 2013 I took the natural next step to become an accredited Meditation Teacher and in the following year I was incredibly honoured to be asked to be a Meditation Teacher Trainer for the British School of Meditation. I now head up their South West regional training centre and I love supporting people with their professional development.

My boyfriend, who had supported me throughout M.E., became my husband and we now have two amazing boys. I still play in a band and can often be found playing festivals every year. Life is still busy and is full of everyday ups and downs and twists and turns, but I can navigate all the changes by utilising everything I have learnt along the way. I know how important it is to look after myself so I can help support those who need my help.

I have also learned to live in the moment rather than worry about the future, or get sad about the past. I am comfortable with my own emotions as well as the emotions of those around me. I am not living each day consumed with fear so I no longer call myself the "born worrier". I treat myself with kindness and I do not feel the need to people-please any more. I live life on a set of principles which are based on the things I have learned along the way.

I am sharing a few of these here as my top tips for growth:

- Rather than pushing away negative emotions, or feeling fearful of the emotions, choose to sit with them and feel them for a moment. By doing this, you can dissipate the fear around the emotions. Be aware of yourself going into the story around the emotion, and gently let that wash over you, returning again to the emotion. Remind yourself you are important enough to feel your emotion. See if you can locate the feeling the emotion generates in your body. Now breathe out the feeling and the emotion from your body. Choose to let it go.

- Instead of focusing on what is wrong in life, just for this moment focus on all the things that are right. It doesn't have to be anything big; it can be the small things. Maybe you could focus your gratitude on the breath you breathe, or on how great it is to be in your body and experience life. Perhaps you could be grateful for even the smallest of actions from family or friends – this can all be helpful to your day. You could also focus on all the wonderful things in your life which help it to flow better, such as your car, computer and phone (we often curse them when they go wrong). You could marvel at all the aspects of nature on your doorstop too.

- Worry can come from not trusting the process of life so your mind may be speaking to you from a fearful place. If you are worrying, you are falsely believing you are protecting yourself. But worry is a story you are creating with your mind and is not based on facts. Worrying is fiction. Instead you can use one of the following techniques:

  o "Worry, worry", and breathe it out. This way, you are acknowledging the worry, but choosing to let it go

  o About turn: you can take my worry and give it a happy ending.

  o Instead of focusing on the fears, you could write down all the possible solutions to the worries

I have the quote *"We don't see things as they are, we see things as we are"* by Anais Nin, on a blackboard in my kitchen. It is an everyday reminder of the bigger picture to every situation. Being told at the age of 26 I was going to be poorly for the rest of my life was not the truth, it was just one perspective at that time. I am so grateful I chose to view life through a new and improved lens.

Sarah Presley is a Meditation Teacher Trainer and Reiki Master Teacher based in Bristol, UK.

An externally accredited Meditation Teacher Trainer with the British School of Meditation, she loves to provide quality professional development. Sarah brings various levels of meditation courses to her local community, schools and businesses. She loves to support individuals with their personal development through reiki offering treatments and training in the various degrees.

Sarah's first book will aim to help people to make friends with themselves by using the life changing techniques of meditation. She will provide know-how on how to meditate and how these techniques help people to gain a new and improved perspective on their lives.

www.sarahpresley.co.uk

THE OPEN ROAD
Sue Williams

Today I take the wheel.
No longer wait for other clowns
To critique the ups and downs
Of my life.

I am the driver, I seize the wheel,
I pay for the gas; I seal the deal.
I embrace the freedom of the open road,
No longer back-seat driver allowed to goad.

I turn the switch, I select the station,
Which words or music suit my destination.
I choose the direction, I plan the route,
Playfully, I give my horn a toot!

Straight to the point, or meandering free,
Mine is the path that seizes opportunity.
At a crossroads, I read the signs,
I may decide not to travel in straight lines.

Occasionally, I stop, pick up a fellow traveller,
Chat, banter, share the load, help to unravel her
Golden dreams. Sisterhood often means
Greater success in our shared hopes and schemes.

Back at the wheel, I travel on alone,
With all the resources, I claim as my own.
My inner tool box will carry me far,
I am the owner; I choose the car.

I am the driver, I take the wheel,
I travel in whichever direction I feel.

214

BEING IN ALIGNMENT
~ *Maggie Prestidge*

"We can realise in a moment that something isn't feeling good and is out of alignment with who we are." Maggie Prestidge

I have walked that pathway, and I am now putting what I have learnt into this book in the hope that whoever needs it finds it at just the right time.

Putting the old programming hat on for a minute, I recognise that with the closure of a profitable business that I had started from scratch, along with the materialistic lifestyle it created, turned me from a successful professional into a victim. I can see that now. Being out of tune with unfulfilling work is energy draining; in my case, causing the body to fall apart.

Being out of alignment led me to make some impractical decisions, including taking on bigger premises, increasing staffing, a luxury car, designer jewellery and a boyfriend who served me no purpose. I did not take time to rest; instead I was always on the go, rushing everywhere, working crazily busy hours.

However, knowing as I do now that everything has a reason and that the Universe is acting in our favour, takes away the judgement and blame I once put upon myself in creating my story. Being out of alignment created an opportunity for me to come into alignment. I decided to close the door on a business with a six-figure turnover, yet which created so many negative and unpleasant circumstances for me. By doing so, I opened up a doorway to heaven.

My new understanding that from an adverse situation comes good was inspired in me at that time by Jan, a Spiritual Mechanic living in Hove, Sussex, who supported me. Those words of inspiration have stayed with me ever since.

I had been busy carrying around judgements on how it "should" be to run a "successful" business. I thought I had to keep growing the business, making it bigger and better, taking on more tasks, clients and financial investments. But by doing so, I was allowing the essence of who I really was to fade away.

My successful business was not congruent with how I felt inside. I was continually putting on a smile and covering up fears and worries, hoping they would disappear. In a way, they did.

Yet I was neglecting the positive in me, and my ability to receive. I was shutting down, crying myself to sleep before waking up, exhausted, to start over again. I was evoking the Law of Attraction at its finest; for example, I used to dread receiving bills in the post. So, what happened?

A large request for taxes arrived from the Inland Revenue as the business had made substantial profits in 2006.

A downturn in the UK market followed by the "crash" meant that the money set aside to pay this bill was used to see the business through the downturn. The said bill therefore, remained unpaid!

Having sought expert advice, I took the difficult decision to put the business into liquidation; one of the hardness experiences of my life. It is way up there with divorce (yes, I have done that one as well!).

Although the signs were right in front of me, still my old pattern of "keep on going" prevailed. A very big sign that I should disband the business and downsize confronted me on my return from a holiday, when six therapists handed in their notice within one week! This left four empty practitioner rooms.

However, me being me back then, I went in search of anyone who offered a therapy, so I could fill the rooms, soothe my ego and receive rent. This was not in alignment with my highest self, even though I acknowledge I did engage some very good therapists!

I believe that in treading the path of this life there is no such thing as bad luck. We make things happen, we have a purpose, a mission in this life, and if we are out of alignment something will happen to put us back on track. This is certainly what happened to me.

In being out of alignment we get confused, we think differently, and attack becomes our chosen form of defence. If you pay attention, you'll observe this in others. Instead of retaliating, stop and wonder what is going on for them that makes them feel that way.

I invite you to get curious and view situations differently. It is possible for us to approach things in a new way, and to achieve good returns whilst being the best we can be. This, in turn, leads us to make the right choices at the right time.

There is no such thing as failure, unless we choose to see it that way, which is coming from a place of judgement. It's about our preferences and actively choosing the best ways for our lifestyle to be in alignment.

I choose to be happy, and I now live in the north of Spain, enjoying the sunshine with two cats and a dog; blending in with nature and listening to the sounds of the birds. I allow myself to do work appropriate for who I am. Therefore, at the time of writing this I am working randomly on projects which find me, and with people who light my fire, whilst taking time to meander, potter and be with friends who inspire and uplift me.

A good mechanic makes thing work well. Mastering me and being my own best mechanic has taken practice, but then I had a good mechanic to learn from too, which helps!

When we believe good things can happen, they will. Here are some techniques which are tried and tested on myself and which I have found work quickly. I would love you to join in, feel good and be in alignment!

EXERCISES:

A dose of feel-good

1. Wake up in the morning slowly, stretching unhurriedly (observe cats – they are very clever at it!). Have a dialogue with yourself about how the day will work for you. Ask what needs to happen to make it work in your favour. Picture how it might happen.

2. When you feel good about something, say to yourself "I like this", "I want more of it". Watch as each thing unfolds and be grateful. Saying "thank you" is sending out a positive statement to the Universe.

3. Take time to be still. Stillness allows for good things to come in. When you still the mind, peace comes in, which allows those droplets of inspiration and intuition to enter.

Maggie Prestidge lives on the Isle of Wight and enjoys its quaintness. She spends her days junk journaling, and being relaxed. She offers the crafting community an opportunity to own ethically sourced Indian saree fabric for their creativity. See the glorious colours & fabrics at Facebook: https://www.facebook.com/beachandsaree Be inspired by the creations made by her design team partner Ali on her YouTube channel: *The Cockney Crafter.*

219

WOW-FULL WOMEN, IGNITE YOUR LIGHT!
Sue Williams

Two hundred women;
closeted in creative conference room.
Oh, how their divine energy can lift the gathering gloom;
Experienced outside in rampant rain; rising flood.
Inside, spirituality at work, inspiring genuine good!
Surrender to an aura of positive, purposeful intent,
Swelled by chatter and laughter; the atmosphere, rent
With the amazing energetic alchemy
Of love and acceptance, true feminine essence
of you and me.

Inspired; yet subtly stirs up your "stuff"
Observe and learn, what makes you feel rough?
There's a yearning for emotional release from deep inside,
No longer glorious inner goddess given space to hide!
Doubts, regrets, dread and fear,
Let each one out, welcome them here.
For, they are ready to heal and go,
Allowing authentic inner spirit to shine, and grow!

As we say farewell to this joy-filled event: "Ignite",
Which turned up the volume of spiritual light,
Wow-full women, awakening to live their dreams!
Way forward for this world, it seems;
Dalai Lama got it right,
Will be western women shining bright!

WHEN THE GLOBE BREAKS
~ *Jo Roberts*

'You are a child of the universe, no less than the trees and the stars. You have a right to be here. And whether or not it is clear to you, no doubt the universe is unfolding as it should.' Max Ehrmann

Trauma changes us. It doesn't just affect our mood, our opinions; it changes the very fabric of who we are. Like a physical wound which heals and leaves its scars, so too does a trauma to the mind, to the spirit, to the soul.

Pick up a snow globe and shake it so hard that it almost breaks. The scene becomes obscured though the torrent of power which rages through, but once the seismic waves have stopped the flakes eventually fall. To the casual observer the scene hasn't changed, it has returned to its 'normal self' - but look closer and the flakes can never again be settled in the same way.

And if the globe is shaken again and again and again sometimes it does break and the effects are obvious to see, a change in how someone looks, how someone acts, how someone can cope with life. Sometimes we manage to 'fix' the cracks, glue back the shattered pieces and sometimes these repairs become so neat, so unseen that they become forgotten, hidden from public view.

The cause of such cataclysmic shifts will be as different and unique as we are; a brain injury, a life-threatening illness, war, abuse, a road accident, or bereavement. And like the shattered globe, it's coping with wave after wave of pain, of shock, of grief that can eventually break us.

November 26th 2015

My friend Wyn, calmly calls nine-nine-nine. "*Ambulance please …. Excessive bleeding, miscarriage.*"

I lean my head onto my arm, and hold onto the side of the bath; knees and feet pooled in a congealing sea of blood. I've been here alone for hours, determined that all would be okay, that I could look after myself. I'm fourteen weeks pregnant, but not pregnant – at least not any more. Development stopped many weeks ago, 'No heartbeat.' Yet somehow the message didn't filter through to my body; I continued to have swollen boobs, nausea, a bloated stomach… The placenta must have kept on growing and now, although I don't know it, it is stuck. My life blood, quite literally, draining away.

The order of things

I love being outside, I love the breeze on my face and the green hills of home but like many of us, I have struggled with my mental health. My mum died when I was in my early twenties and often with a smile on my face, a mask unwittingly plastered in place, I got on with living; launching myself into new adventures, searching perhaps, but for what, I didn't know.

I'd grown up knowing that my mum had miscarried my twin, but I'd never asked many questions.

After she went it was too late to ask her and somehow, hidden inside there was a part of me that just wasn't complete.

In 2005 I met Nat. Love blossomed and despite many challenges we made a welcoming and loving home and often his young son, my (almost) stepson came to stay.

But gradually there were increasing tensions; I felt stuck, with an unfulfilling work life and no real sense of purpose. The pull of motherhood, once suppressed and dormant began to raise her head and I could no longer ignore her. However, being diagnosed with unexplained infertility in April 2015, the day before I turned forty, wasn't quite how we'd envisaged things going. And when we were told we weren't eligible to receive IVF through the NHS — the reality of our journey fell over us, like a blanket, slowly smothering.

I began researching elsewhere, and in so doing discovered a whole new world — an uplifting, holistic and fundamentally different way of experiencing life. Through meditation and energy work, I was unwittingly being equipped to deal with what was to come and amazingly I fell pregnant that September.

For a few short weeks I was truly happy. The challenges, the stresses; they just fell away. I was pregnant. I was somebody's mum. For two months my whole being was devoted to growing our baby-to-be; my purpose ahead of

223

me. I was fascinated by this magical development and they became as much a part of me as my own beating heart.

But on October 28th 2015, a bright sunny day in Cumbria; my little world started its inward collapse. Attending a routine medical appointment, I walked into Barrow Hospital, ten weeks pregnant and as content with my life as I ever had been. Sometime later I was walking away – and nothing would ever be the same again. I'd had an impromptu scan. No heart beat could be found; and where there should have been a tiny pulsing life, there was nothing.

How could I not have known? It turned out development had stopped at only 6 and a half weeks — nothing in an average life. For nearly a month I'd felt more and more pregnant; nausea raising its head, tiredness too — and yet as I talked to our baby-to-be - they had quietly slipped away. A conception we had longed for had entered our lives in a month we hadn't thought possible and left without us knowing.

About a month I waited in limbo, willing the doctors to be wrong; concocting any number of elaborate, desperate reasons as to how my baby would still be coming. Then at fourteen weeks, in the privacy of my own bathroom my body was finally trying to relinquish all that it had fought so hard to protect. Contractions had been washing over me for hours, pain coming in waves, clots passing and then brief lulls. Eventually the pain stopped and my body was desperate to rest. But the blood kept coming. I was calm, too calm, and somewhere deep within my inner survival I knew I needed help.

November 26th 2015
An ambulance comes, whisks me away, sirens blaring, lights on; my safe haven gone.

"Tachycardic … amber alert," says the paramedic into her radio.

When we arrive at Lancaster hospital I am immediately surrounded by the NHS's finest. *Wham!* A driving force of pain shoots through me as one doctor tries unsuccessfully to release the blockage.

An uncontrollable thunder escapes from my previously quiet voice at the onslaught of her hand inside me and then a shot of ketamine suspends life as I know it. I trip out big time and my response to this hideous drug leaves me terrified. I come around, not knowing *what* I am, let alone who or where am.

Four pints of heated blood later, an emergency anaesthetic and finding myself holding the hand of yet another wonderful medical personnel, I am cocooned under a warm air-filled blanket.

That night I have the strongest sense that my spirit daughter is watching over me. Not the soul I'd been pregnant for, but his sister.

She comes to me as a light filled, angelic being and she reassures me that her brother is resting, recovering well from our shared trauma.

I am flipped out – between this loving, comfortable spirit world and the cold hard reality of earthly sorrow I make it through my first night, deeply sad, internally hollow; but alive.

The next afternoon, weak but capable of showering myself; of washing away the pungency, I am allowed home. I have some delayed reaction though; to the shock, the ketamine or most likely the anaesthetic. My torso is in agony, my neck stiff and my words miss-formed. I just want the world to stop. A different hospital and a less than sympathetic doctor add to my distress. We never do find out the exact cause, but it's as if my body and mind, exhausted, have just imploded.

Unable to cope anymore my snow-globe cracks open and I sink to my lowest depths. I've lost my baby-to-be and in the process I've all but lost the hope of myself. I can't comprehend life in this new forever changed world, and my body, its new blood merging with the old, feels numb.

The Snowflakes Will Fall
As the snowflakes settled, as the physical cracks started to heal, I gradually learned to operate within my changed life. But in trying to heal the inner pain, in coping with the re occurring trauma; in starting to live a new life, I no

longer fitted into the imprint of the old one.

And no matter how much I resisted, how much I raged there was one more globe breaking blow waiting to happen — and in January 2017 my fragile life smashed into another million pieces when Nat told me he was leaving our relationship.

This second irreversible change held one bigger thought. Despite my shock, my inner collapse, I knew one thing; I've survived the worst that has ever happened in my life, so somehow, I know that I can, and will, survive this.

Learning to live and love my new life

And I did survive. Somehow, with the love and support of others, I glued the shattered pieces and built a new life. A close friend recently said, "It's good to see you back to your old self again."

But that *old self* belongs to the past, to a life which is no longer mine. In her place is an evolving self, a more truth-filled self; thankful for all her experiences.

Of course, I look the same (well, maybe a few more grey hairs). I likely sound the same, but my take on life has changed through my fertility journey. Even some of the language I use to express myself is different. Energy, spirit, meditation are all daily experiences within my life, as I recognise and honour all that has gone before.

It is said that time heals – but I believe that it's what we do with that time, which offers the true healing. Grieving, consciously learning to let go, spending time doing things we love, reflecting, challenging self-beliefs, looking after ourselves and seeing exquisite beauty; these are some of the ways in which we heal.

The sun does not shine every day, sometimes the winds rage and the seas crash. Some days I live with constant inner noise; building, screaming. Sometimes I still wonder what it would be like to step off this earth and many days I still cry, as some welled up emotion tumbles out. But I know this is important too. It's healing taking place deep inside.

Not long after my miscarriage I made a promise to myself, to the universe, to my baby in spirit. If I wasn't ready to die, then surely, I must find a way to live. I promised myself that I would do *what* I could *when* I could. It isn't always easy, but little by little my steps have become bigger, my sorrow less and my joy greater.

My life is no longer in crisis. I'm excited to be finding a new 'normal' and I am learning to love myself more deeply than I have ever done before. I have come to believe that the universe gives us what we need, not necessarily what we *think* we want.

For whatever reason, my life needed shaking up; I needed taking to my limits, so that I could build a new tomorrow. I am still on my journey to parenthood; but the universe *is* unfolding as it should. I no longer feel stuck.

I have experienced maternal love deep inside and I understand the power of holding intention, of raising vibration and most of all of loving this world enough to hold myself accountable for the promise I made.

When you need a little help to trust that the universe is unfolding as it should:

1. Make a Thankful list

Every night for almost a year I wrote down ten things I was thankful for that day. The cumulative healing power was amazing.

2. Transform unhelpful thoughts to uplifting energy

Identify three emotions you are experiencing and then name the opposite.

Tired, Sad and *Frustrated*
could become
Energised, Content and *Patient*.

Repeat these new words lovingly (internally or out-loud).

This tends to have an immediate impact on me – but I use it carefully, so that uncomfortable feelings can still be expressed.

3. Journal a stream of consciousness

My most memorable emergency use was on a train. I felt
exceptionally overwhelmed and vulnerable.
I sat in my seat, pulled out my note book and soothed my
inner panic with every word I wrote.

Jo Roberts hails originally from South West England.
She has since made her home within the fabulous
Cumbrian landscape. Currently writing her first novel,
One Step Forwards, she draws on experiences of grief, joy
and of learning to live again. *When the Globe Breaks* is a
massive step on her own journey of transformation and is
shared with love.

YOUR SIGNATURE SUCCESS STORY
Sue Williams

Join us, celebrate, before it gets too late!
Don't allow enthusiasm to abate,
Success is there for you to take,
Please don't leave it too near your wake,
Really something to contemplate…

What makes you truly unique?
The way you walk, or how you speak?
Wisdom and knowledge shared in a book,
The daring deeds, the risks you took?

Raising a boisterous family;
A high-powered career; high visibility?
Do you feel you've reached your peak?
Or more fulfilment dare to seek?

When do you experience playfulness, fun?
Are there tall tales still to be spun?
A new adventure, mountain to climb?
Perhaps you're thinking "It's my time"?

We all have our signature moves,
Our distinctive rhythm, beat and grooves,
We each define our own success,
Perhaps by reclaiming, re-naming our "mess!"

What are your ingredients for Signature Success?
How best with the world your gifts express?
Now is the time to claim your feminine power,
And into the world, your true essence shower.

Capture your story, uncover your true voice,
How you employ it, that's your own choice.
Whether in family, community, a book, or on screen,
Now is the time for you to shine, be seen!

SOMETHING HAPPENED TO ME
~ *Andrea Tickle*

"It's not what you go through that defines you; you can't help that. It's what you do AFTER you've gone through it that really tests who you are." - Kwame Floyd

On 9 May 2008 something happened to me. Some might say something for the worse, but I wholeheartedly believe it was for the better... and I'll tell you why. At the age of 26 I found myself "stuck in a rut". Living on the borders of London with my sister, young and free of responsibilities, I thought my life would be exciting.

Unfortunately, I was hugely unfulfilled. In a desperate search to change my life, I landed myself a job in Australia. The flights were booked, but the proposed move to Australia never felt "real" and I guess it's because it was never meant to be...

One sunny Friday morning, I set off in my car for work. I remember putting homemade soup in a thermos flask for lunch and listening to Radio 2. What I don't remember is having a head-on collision with an HGV lorry and being air-lifted to the Royal London Hospital.

My injuries were serious. I had fractured both bones in my right leg (the femur and tibia), the big bone in my left leg, every bone in my right arm, my right collarbone, a vertebra in my neck, a few ribs and a couple of bones in my foot and hand. Thirteen in total! But that wasn't the

233

main concern for the doctors. I'd also suffered a pneumothorax (punctured lung) and ruptured my small intestine and colon.

I spent just under a week in intensive care and three months in hospital. My memories of hospital are some of the most traumatic, and I can still feel overwhelmed not by what happened to me, but what my family had to stand by and witness. I had two external metal cages on my legs, and without the use of my right arm and bandaged burns on the left arm, I relied on help for everything.

My family were always there for me. Even when I was in intensive care with a machine helping me to breathe, they made a chart with all the letters of the alphabet so that I could point and communicate with them. I remember spelling out "I L O V E Y O U".

So, time passed, and I began to feel safe going out in a wheelchair. My mum and I went to live with my grandmother in Kent, as she has a bungalow. As I got better, my granddad and I would pass each other in the hallway with our Zimmer frames and smile! After nine months in a wheelchair, I was happy to be a Zimmer chick! My mum and I could now move back to the family home in Coventry with my dad and younger brother. After all, there's only so long you can leave two men alone in a house!

And so, the long road to recovery continued. My time was taken up with hospital appointments, physiotherapy, chiropractic and many other healing therapies. I went to art classes, pottery workshops and spent my time cooking, sleeping and allowing my body to heal.

I had on-going problems with my legs that meant I needed more surgery. Strangely, I looked forward to the upcoming surgery date with a sense of hope and nervous anticipation. I believed that the surgery would fix my problems. Unfortunately, the surgery didn't work out as planned. Doctors told me they would perform another operation, but I was feeling the effects of repeated doses of anaesthetic and I wanted to move on with my life. By this point I had met a wonderful man called James.

James and I met at a mutual friend's fancy dress birthday party. I was dressed as Minnie Mouse and he was Dennis the Menace! We spent fun times together, but there were hard times too. Despite all of my scars, tiredness and inability to walk very far, James wined, dined and romanced me. But more importantly, he held my hand through it all and looked after me.

James and I wanted to move in together, and I wanted a job. I had qualified as a chiropractor in 2004, but after my accident I wasn't sure I would be well enough to return to this physical job. However, my passion for chiropractic was at an all-time high. It was my chiropractic colleagues that got me out of that wheelchair and walking again.

The power of chiropractic really shouldn't be underestimated. The multiple physiotherapists that I saw tried their best, but they didn't have the time to properly address all my injuries. Chiropractors look at the person as a whole, and treat their emotional as well as the physical needs.

So, I found myself thinking – chiropractic is not just a job, it is my way of life. It has given me life! I felt that as I had the skill and training, it was a gift and I must share it to help all those people with back pain, neck pain, elbow, knee, wrist pain… all the symptoms I had experienced.

I was in the perfect position to set up a chiropractic service knowing what people really want when they're in pain. Someone to listen, understand and provide a high-quality, hands-on treatment, that addresses ALL the problems. I didn't want to be rushed and I needed additional advice on things like exercise – what was best for me, considering my injuries?

Happily, I now have my own successful chiropractic business, where the emphasis is on the unique needs of the patient. I strive to give every person the first-class treatment and attention to detail that I wanted.

Moving back to Coventry was daunting (and a bit depressing compared to the dream of moving to Australia), but little did I know that I was entering the happiest time of my life. I'm surrounded by my family, I've made contact again with my primary school friends, I have a fantastic business helping people and, above all else, I married the man of my dreams on 31 March 2012!

This is a very short story of my experiences over the last four years. My patients often say to me "You should write a book." I was delighted to be asked to write a chapter for this book; I have an inner voice pushing me to share the message that everything happens for a reason. My experiences have given me a greater understanding of pain, and have driven me to help as many people as I can.

Finding your purpose in life is truly satisfying. I want to spread the word of living a life where we seek "not to sweat the small stuff". Belief is everything. Even when I was lying trapped in a hospital bed, I imagined myself running through the park. I believed I would make a full recovery and despite the set-backs, I did. Every day that I wake up, get out of bed and put my foot on the ground, I am grateful that I can walk. I'm even more grateful to have a second opportunity in life to make a difference.

EXERCISES:

1. Set goals that inspire and excite you. Give the goal a set time frame, so that you have something to work towards. It might be helpful to set mini-goals, if necessary, to help you achieve the main goal.

I find it useful to rule out time in my diary to do the task. Treat the time like you would another appointment. You wouldn't miss a dentist appointment, so honour yourself and keep any appointments that you make with yourself. Another thing I found helpful with goal setting is not to worry if or when, your goal changes. Goals just give us something to work towards, but they don't have to be set in stone.

2. Make a decision without worrying whether it is the right decision. You can spend a lot of time thinking, analysing and wondering whether you are travelling down the right path. I recommend reading a "Who Moved my Cheese" by Dr Spencer Johnson. It's a short story which highlights that those who make decisions more quickly can suss out faster whether they are on the right track!

3. Practise being open to people and opportunities. It is easy to judge someone or something before getting to know them or finding out more. Some time ago I was asked out on a date – the old me would have declined, thinking "We haven't got anything in common. There's no point." I'm glad the new me was open to possibilities because that first date led to a wonderful marriage!

Andrea Tickle is a Doctor of Chiropractic. She helps people to enjoy good health by finding and correcting the root cause of their problems. Find out more at www.greystonehealthyliving.com

FAITH
Hannah Imogen Jones

I have faith that the sun will rise each day
I have faith that the young will laugh and play
I have faith that love always will show me the way
I have faith in my loved ones and I.

I have faith that there's more to this lifetime of ours
I have faith that believing will soon open doors
I have faith that this cosmos is my home and yours
I have faith that there's magic and beauty in store.

I have faith in the testing decisions I'll make
I have faith I can separate real from fake
I have faith there'll be changes and changes I'll make
I have faith I'll have chances and chances I'll take.

I have faith in the past and will have no regrets
I have faith in my dreams, they will be achieved yet
I have faith in each dawn and the truth it begets
I have faith that my actions will still make amends.

I have faith there's a reason that I am here now
I have faith there are many things that I can do
I have faith my experience and wisdom will show
I have faith there are many great things that I know.

I have faith in my courage and faith in my strength
I have faith that sweet love will prevail in the end
I have faith in my family and faith in my friends
I have faith that the beauty of life never ends.

I have faith I will shine through the darkest of nights
I have faith in the power and beauty of light
I have faith that sweet freedom is my divine right
I have faith that my soul will be raised to flight.

FROM SEXUAL SLAVERY
TO SPIRITUAL AWAKENING
~ *Lisa Turner*

"No matter how free your body is, unless your mind is free you are a psychic slave." Dr Lisa Turner

This story is shocking. Whenever I tell it, people are shocked. It's shocking for two reasons.

Firstly, when people look at me, they see a successful business woman, in a great marriage, with a confident daughter, all living in a nice home. I'm living the life I dreamt of. They see a happy person. But being a happy person is at odds with everything they've been told about how someone who's been through what I've been through "should" be like.

Apparently, I should be filled with neuroses, with phobias and panic attacks. I shouldn't be able to experience intimacy, let alone sustain a happy relationship or experience a satisfying sex life. I shouldn't be able to hold down a job, let alone run a multi-six-figure business. People find this astonishing.

The other reason people are shocked by my story is, because, quite frankly, it's shocking!

What I experienced was so far removed from what is considered a "normal" (or at least common) childhood that jaws drop as I share my story. As each successive stage is unveiled, they become more and more intrigued as to how such a thing could happen. What were the adults in my life thinking? How could anyone behave like that? And the most common question of all is: "How did you escape?"

So, let's start at the beginning.

I grew up in Australia. My parents emigrated when I was little more than a baby and all I had known was bright blue skies, warm Christmases, open spaces and open minds. Australia and my parents were liberal in their thinking, accepting in their views and most of all loving. I was loved, happy and normal. Not perfect, but normal.

At the age of 12 I took private guitar lessons with the school music teacher. Over the next few months and years he seduced my psyche, my ego and took over my life. I spent more and more time with him, neglecting my friends. He became the centre of my world. He ensured this. I was 13 when he first attempted penetrative sex. I was 14 when he succeeded. I was 15 when he convinced me and my parents to send me with him to England. The original plan was for me to spend only a few short months there, to learn more about music and experience the country of my birth.

Over a period of months, he charmed my parents into believing that this short visit would be perfect for my education, after which I would return. Of course, I never did.

Over the next five years, until I escaped, I experienced the systematic torture and destruction of my psyche. I became a psychic slave to his happiness, and his misery. I ceased to exist as a person. I had no desires of my own, no interests, no hobbies, and no sense of self. Over the years it had been eroded. I was left with nothing.

He made it very clear that I was responsible for his happiness. In simple terms this is a co-dependent relationship. "I can't live/be happy/survive/cope without you." Although this might sound like love and forms the basis of the lyrics for many love songs, it's actually a prison sentence. I'd been brought up to be kind and considerate of others' feelings. I wanted others to be happy.

What I didn't realise was that I was making myself unhappy for the sake of his happiness. Indeed, often he would punish me if I was happy or laughed, with shouting, moodiness, and mild violence. He would punish me for crying too. I stopped showing my feelings.

Eventually I stopped feeling. I simply second-guessed what he wanted me to feel, always glancing at him for clues as to what emotion to display. My focus was so on his happiness that it became impossible to tell where his desires ended and mine began. So enslaved was my mind that from the outside, to my friends and family, I looked happy.

My freedom was severely restricted. I was allowed to go to school, but not allowed any extracurricular activities. I wasn't allowed friends. I didn't speak about any friends I had. My school mates thought I was living in bliss. After all, wasn't I living the life many schoolgirls dreamt of, living with my boyfriend in a flat with no rules from parents? They thought I must be so free. Little did they know how much like a prison my life was.

He controlled everything: the grocery budget, the heating, when we ate, slept what we watched on TV. It was made clear that I was to cook for him, and he told me what to cook. If I ate something that had not been authorised before he returned from work there was hell to pay. He would shout and tell me how selfish I was. He made a particular point of usually telling me how no one else would ever have me. He would ration meals saying that as I had already eaten, I wouldn't want any. He rarely needed to use physical violence as by then I was so compliant.

His anger was enough to control me.

He controlled the sexual relationship. Whereas my school friends imagined that we were at it every night, the truth was very different. He would go for months without touching me. I quickly learned never to attempt to instigate sex. The first time I reached out to him on the couch whilst watching TV he screamed that I was a slut and perverted, and that I was so unattractive that no one would want me.

On the rare occasions he did instigate sex it was brutal. I was little more than an object to be used. There was no love, no touching and no connection. He would not speak to me and he didn't touch me, except to force himself into me.

Other than school and grocery shopping I lived as a house prisoner. I only did things he permitted, things he chose. I was his slave. But he did not build physical walls. He built a psychic prison cell. He trained me to only think of pleasing him, and to desperately avoid displeasing him. He did not need to force his will on me, so completely had he eroded any sense of me that I had had: body, mind and soul. I had become a slave to his psyche, his mind.

What people often find shocking is not only that I stayed and that I stayed for so long, but that I managed to escape. The question people most ask is "How did you get out?"

It wasn't instant or quick. My freedom revealed itself slowly in a sequence of fortunate events. Just as he had slowly but surely enslaved me, without realising it, I was slowly but surely taking the steps to freedom.

The most significant step was when I began to realise that he didn't know everything. He was wrong sometimes. As I moved on in my schooling to the time where my studies of maths were greater than his, a discussion revealed that I knew more about maths than he did. I was suddenly shocked to realise this. That seemingly insignificant moment planted the seed of realisation that maybe there were other things that he didn't know about too, or even that he was wrong about!

I began to question. I questioned that he knew what was best for me. I began to question that he knew what I should and should not do or be or like. I realised that some of the things I believed I liked I had only chosen in an attempt to please him. Actually, I didn't like them!

I started to question everything. Only in my mind at first, but this questioning led me to believe that there was a way out. This belief was what triggered me to leave.

It eventually took about six months to summon up the resolve and inner strength for me to finally leave. I worked every holiday I could, doing admin work and data entry, saving every penny until I had enough to move into a small, sordid bedsit in a crowded shared house. And it was bliss.

It took many, many more years for me to fully recover my sense of self. My psyche was so programmed to only think of him, it took many years before I could fully think of myself.

And now, through my belief, I live a life of freedom. I am no longer a slave to anyone's happiness. What is even more shocking for many people is that I am not a psychic slave even to what others call "real". I choose my

245

happiness. I choose not to allow circumstances to dictate my options or to narrow my options. I understand at a deep level that the universe is always conspiring to support us, even if it doesn't always feel like that in the moment.

Most importantly, I believe that my mind is free and that I will never be a psychic slave again. Not only am I not a slave to any other person. I'm also not a psychic slave to circumstances, experiences, and my past.

Perhaps for some this last point is the most shocking of all. That anyone can be free from pain from the past, so ingrained is the belief that pain from the past will stay with us forever. I have learned that pain can be released and we can be free.

EXERCISES:

1: Power Breath Meditation
This power breath meditation is known as "HA breathing". For best results, practice it for 10 minutes a day. It will energise your body, increase your inner strength, intuition, personal power, balance emotions and clear your mind and thoughts.

Begin by sitting upright and relax.

Take a deep breath in through your nose.

Make sure you breathe into the diaphragm so that your stomach moves in and out.

Breathe out through your mouth and as you do so, slightly constrict your throat so the air comes out slowly. If you are doing it right it should make a hissing or HAAA sound, like air coming out of a tyre. It's very like whispering.

As you breathe out your stomach comes slowly in. Your breath expands your stomach and diaphragm on the in-breath.

The out-breath should be at least twice as long as the in-breath.

Keep breathing out until you have emptied your lungs. When you have breathed all the way out, take another deep breath in through your nose.

During HA breathing you may notice that your eyes may begin to water. This is common and perfectly normal and natural. HA breathing increases the amount of the water element (covered in depth in another course), and watering eyes is a sign that balance is being restored to your body. If you practice HA breathing regularly you will find it stops, indicating that balance has been achieved.

For a free instant access to a guided meditation to meet your higher self, go to www.meetyourhigherself.com

2: Where are your power leaks?

Answer these questions to increase your self-awareness about any power leaks you might have.

Where do you not do your best?

What events or situations make you feel better than others?

When and with whom do you allow yourself to be intimidated?

What events in the past have made you feel disempowered?

In what ways do you sabotage yourself (or others)?

Where do you think of yourself as superior to others? Where do you HAVE to be better than others?

Where do you agree to keep the peace?

Where do you disagree to?

What do you avoid?

What do you deny?

What are you pretending not to know?

In what ways are you not physically powerful? What do illnesses or physical ailments "do" to you?

List three ways you intend to change as a result of this.

3: Reconnect with your physical body

When your body communicates with you do you listen? Do you know how your body sends you messages? Do you ever "answer"? You're certainly familiar with some; you probably know when you are hungry, or hot or cold. But you can communicate in a way that's far more sophisticated and exquisite, by building a relationship with your body.

The way in which your body communicates is different for different people. For some it is sensations, tingling, heat, cold, or vibrations. For others they may hear sounds, or even "little voices". Other people get images, or flashes of inspiration about what their body needs.

Lying down or sitting comfortably with your eyes closed, take a moment to settle and turn inward. Consciously and actively send a message to your body, in whatever way feels right for you. Start by "asking" your body to communicate, or just say "hello" to it. You might want to apologise for not communicating consciously with it before.

Let your body know that you would like to have a really good relationship with it. Allow whatever answer comes to arrive in your awareness, just as a knowing.

Start doing this process on a regular basis. When you are under a lot of pressure during a busy period, let your body know how long you will be making increased demands on it. Make a deal with your body, e.g. "If you keep going, allowing me to push and work you hard until Saturday, I will allow you a whole day off." Make sure you keep your end of the deal – or your body will not trust you.

If your body gets sick, with a cold say, go inside and ask it why it got sick. Then ask it what it needs you to do to make it better as quickly as possible.

As you build a relationship with your body, and keep your promises to it, you will find that you get sick less, become stronger, and better able to cope.

Take time to move your body, and notice how it feels to move. So right now, stand up and start to move. Keep moving. That's about it really. You can put some music on if this helps, select some that is inspiring or relaxing.

We won't call it dancing, as we might be tempted to impose judgements about what constitutes dancing. The purpose is to get moving. You will find any embarrassment you might feel will quickly go as you start moving and enjoying the movement. Start slowly and gently, perhaps by swaying slightly, or wiggling your fingers. Allow the finger movement to expand upwards into your wrists and then your arms.

Allow your arms to move upwards and outwards, as high, as wide, and at any pace that feels comfortable. Just move.

Try shaking, as an athlete does before their event. Shaking out your legs, arms, and hands; turning your head from side to side, around and around.

When you're ready move your hips and start to move into your spine, flexing it from side to side, and forwards and backwards. Always keeping within the limits of what is physically comfortable for you. You might try skipping or jumping, on the spot or wherever.

Are there any tight places in your body? What kinds of movements ease this, and which make it worse? Notice what kind of movements you enjoy most and keep doing those. Experiment and enjoy.

Now notice what you notice.

Lisa Turner is a renowned visionary, author, channel, and master spiritual teacher, who has shared her proven spiritual technology with over 30,000 spiritual practitioners worldwide. She is creator of a number of proven models that explain our past, predict our future and increase success.

With a PhD in Mathematical Modelling and Aero-acoustics, Lisa made the extraordinary transition from scientist to spiritual teacher through her search to become free of her own past in which she was kept by a paedophile, from the age of 15, as a virtual house prisoner. Her experience now fuels her dedication to freeing minds of others who are enslaved by the illusion of their inner limitations.

Find out more at www.psycademy.com

The Art of Doing Nothing
Sue Williams

There's really no need to strive and fear,
Let it all go, just sit here,
All by yourself, not pressurised, just alone
To avoid interruption, turn off that phone!

You can just be, quietly sit,
Breathing healing energy in, allowing it
Without the need for worry, stress or strain,
All that isn't giving you any gain.

This way you are allowing,
Peace and inner calm
To take the helm.
The ship is silent; your surroundings are balm,
Undulating peacefully on the waves,
Rising and falling, anchored in the deep enclaves
Yet ready to set sail, glide serenely over the water,
Wasn't that the reason why you bought her?

There's no need to use brute force
Once cast adrift, effortlessly she holds her course.
Buoyed up on the balmy sea,
Sails billowing, streamlined, surging cleanly forth,
Doesn't matter whether she's headed south or north.

Just know that when you are ready,
You will float silently forward, steady,
Gently and easily you too will meld into your flow.
So, relax here quietly, drink in this scene,
One so calm, peaceful and serene,
Till once again ready to glide smoothly into life's slip stream.

CREATIVITY AND CONNECTION
~ Sue Williams

"At times our own light goes out and is rekindled by a spark from another person. Each of us has cause to think with deep gratitude of those who have lighted the flame within us." Albert Schweitzer

"Sue, stand up! Stand up! Be bold, be strong,
Your talent, on world's stage, truly does belong!"

I wrote these words early one morning in March 2012. They flowed easily and effortlessly as I typed into my computer, and within ten to fifteen minutes I had completed my poem: Believe! I stared at the words on the screen before me with amazement. I had no idea why my writing was flowing so easily, and felt slightly puzzled, yet elated, that it was!

I was quizzical with good reason. The previous evening, I had participated in yet another coaching session; the latest of many healing and self-development activities that I had enrolled in during recent years. I was continually searching for answers. What was causing me to feel disconnected from others and from a real sense of passion and purpose about the direction of my life?

The previous night's event had been broadcast live. This left me with an underlying sense of apprehension and fear. The all too familiar fear of being judged and found wanting; shame at the thought of being exposed as having nothing valuable to say or offer.

254

From a young age, I began to build a protective shell around myself. Whenever something felt too painful, or stirred up unpleasant emotions, I unwittingly put another defence mechanism in place. In 2008, whilst attending "The Journey" workshop with Brandon Bays, despite following a tried and tested script, I struggled to identify where suppressed emotional pain was stored in my body.

In fact, it seemed almost as if my body didn't exist! I was called up to the stage to be coached individually, having publicly expressed my resentment that the process had not worked for me. When questioned by Brandon Bays, all that I could visualise and sense in my head was a triangle of solid glass. Impenetrable. Keeping me safe. Keeping my capacity for creation and self-expression locked firmly inside, whilst allowing me to observe, dispassionately, these abilities in others…

"Something very terrible must have happened to you as a child," Brandon uttered, compassionately.

When young, I possessed a naïvely optimistic Pollyanna type of personality. It seemed perfectly natural to me that everyone would want the best for each other, to get along, and that everything and everyone would be cushioned in a perpetual place of positivity, peace, harmony and happiness! I was quiet and compliant; I also wanted to please.

I was a sensitive soul. One early memory is of my grandfather taking me home as I was too upset to watch scenes in the film "Moses", when a fire blazed in the bulrushes, threatening to engulf a tiny baby in a wickerwork basket. Increasingly, I found it difficult to cope with strong feelings, gradually "zoning out" when things became too uncomfortable or unpleasant.

I stopped watching the news at around the age of ten as I felt overwhelmed by the constant stories of death and disease. Grim images upset my idealistic view of the world, and I couldn't comprehend the reason for all that hurt and pain. Hearing those stories caused negative thoughts to churn painfully around my mind, and generated a sense of helplessness. Why couldn't I do something to stop this? How could this wonderful, magical world encompass such dreadful experiences?

Until the age of around 12 or 13, I was a compulsive book worm; losing myself in the jolly japes of the Famous Five, Secret Seven and the boarders at Mallory Towers, et al. Yarns in which good always triumphed at the end of the tale, and even the unpopular girls at the school found redemption!

However, once too much realism crept into the books recommended for my age group, I changed. I stopped reading books virtually overnight. Books had been my solace, my own secret world, often experienced under the covers after lights out. Reality was creeping in, and I wasn't ready for it.

Shy and introverted, I was also unable to get in touch with, and express my feelings. Gullibly, I would automatically assume that other people's opinions were correct. When I first entered counselling in my early 20s, the counsellor's words felt like a bolt from the blue. On relating how I had been threatened with a knife by another girl some years before, the counsellor enquired: "Did you never ask yourself whether there might have been something wrong with her?" No, I can honestly say I hadn't. I had routinely assumed that there was something wrong with me!

Even through the solace of writing, I was unable to express my inner feelings. Like many children, I kept a diary for several years. However, when I look back at the entries, they only consisted of bland lists of my daily activities: "Walked to town after school. Watched television. Went to Brownies. Mum made apricot crumble for tea. Had an early night." Mentally, I beat myself up for not having anything more meaningful to say. Self-critical by nature, I constrained myself, and my writing was confined by my own judgements.

Yet, visualise an ideal home life, and mine probably looked just like that image. My parents were always there, providing a stable, safe and secure family environment. However, my mum was a dominant force within the family. A formidable woman, highly intelligent with clear-cut views, the sharp sound of her critical comments would regularly lacerate the peace.

Her internal picture of what a "good" family should be didn't match the reality she experienced! I recall her questioning: "What is wrong with this family, why can't you be like other families?" I puzzled over how other families seemingly gelled so much better than ours.

Not that we mixed much as a family; mum felt too embarrassed for anyone other than very close relatives to visit our house.

Picture, if you will, the chaotic jumble of a typical, slightly messy family home, with the clutter exacerbated by mum's penchant for collectibles and souvenirs of days out; and dad's piles of newspapers, awaiting his attention when he had time.

On occasion, the weight of mum's expectations felt oppressive. When she asked: "Why can't you be more like your cousin?" it was an unanswerable question for me, since my cousin was blond and feminine, whilst I was dark haired and a bit of a tomboy. As with most senseless comparisons, the question stayed with me for decades, going around in my head.

I was the middle child, sandwiched between two brothers who often didn't get on. It was nothing too serious; just two immature boys whose tastes and personalities clashed. I clearly remember once, when another disagreement had erupted out of the blue and I was about to step in, the realisation hit me – there was no point!

Consciously, I chose not to interfere; I sat back until their animosity subsided. Similarly, when my mother berated me for getting on her nerves by laughing (cackling, she called it!) or for not meeting her expectations, I submitted to her will, becoming increasingly quiet and amenable. Meanwhile, my dad, a quiet, gentle man, adopted the approach "anything for a quiet life". He and I regularly faded into the background.

Habitually avoiding conflict, my sense of disconnection grew. I also avoided situations where I might be criticised or hurt. I sought to fit in, not to make waves. I also felt an incredibly strong blood tie with my mother, and wanted to experience the positive feelings that I felt were meant to go alongside this.

In 1990, I attended a personal development course around self-actualisation. My specific goal was to become closer to my mother. Imagine my horror, when role playing in pairs, I heard myself repeating bitterly: "I hate you, I hate you." My partner in the exercise informed me that the look of acute shock on my face was quite a picture! My idealistic illusion that this course would magically provide a simple set of answers was completely shattered.

So, did something terrible happen to me in my childhood? Compared to those who have experienced such nightmares as physical abuse, the early death or loss of a close family member or abandonment, no, I don't believe so. My parents were honest, respectable people who wanted the best for us. When older, I knew that should I lose my job or need practical or material help, my parents would help if they could.

Our family unit merely consisted of a jumble of different personalities, bound by blood, seeking to co-exist as best we could. Yet, we were blissfully unaware of how our individual personality preferences and styles impacted on each other. More importantly, we lacked the skills to talk about our feelings, instead retreating to our own natural qualities as individuals.

As dad "zoned out" in front of the TV after a day at the office, mum would become frustrated by the lack of an equally strong and task-focussed counterpart! (Any DIY or decorating only got done once mum took action!)

Whilst mum's relationship with my dad and the wider family gave her the sense of security she craved, it stifled her individuality and sense of adventure. She had dreams of travelling to Norway, seeing other exciting places, going out and experiencing more of the fun and excitement in life. Returning to work in her fifties rejuvenated her, and brought new friends and focus.

Once I left home, I came to experience periods of contentment juxtaposed with the usual stresses and strains of life; yet I struggled with very low self-esteem. I allowed myself to stay too long in work that I found unrewarding in my 20s.

Although I found more rewarding roles in my 30s and 40s and loyal friendships, I was susceptible to the expectations of others. Increasingly, I would explore different methods of healing, and ways of understanding myself and others; gaining new insights and making gradual progress. Periodically, on courses, or during psychic readings, I was advised to journal; to write whatever materialised, without censure. Yet, repeatedly, I resisted!

Early in 2012, I was again advised to journal by a transformational coach, Natasha, with whom I was working. She was so genuinely excited and enthusiastic when suggesting that I write first thing each morning, that I didn't have the heart to resist any longer.

After only three weeks of daily completing my writing practice, I found words would often flow from my pen in rhyme! This in turn led to poetry. Natasha's enthusiasm had sparked a flame of creativity in me that I was unaware I possessed! Subsequently, her vision of staging an event, "Believe – in your Dreams, Legacy and Power", inspired me to write my poem "Believe!"

About six months later, I revisited my poem. Light finally illuminated the message I had carelessly cast aside once the "Believe!" event had changed in scope. My own words spoke to me from the page. Realisation dawned; I had written those words to shake myself up; to stand up for something I personally believed in. I owed it to myself to express my truest self to the world.

261

Just as my connection with Natasha had awoken my latent creativity, I felt drawn towards connecting with others, seeking to share their insights into belief. Once I let go of my doubts and followed my intuition, I was heartened by how contributions to my "Believe!" book naturally flowed.

What if, by pulling together this anthology others became inspired to share their own hidden gifts and talents more widely with the world? What if in doing so, even one other person found the inspiration to believe in their own talents and gifts? And now, this tantalising possibility which makes the "Believe!" book and the heartfelt contributions to it, truly worthwhile has become reality.

EXERCISES:

1: The morning pages (see Julia Cameron's book: The Artist's Way)

For a minimum of four weeks, commit to getting up half an hour earlier than usual. Spend approximately half an hour each morning writing, long-hand, three sides about anything and everything that comes to you. There is no wrong way to write morning pages. If you feel stuck at any point, it is OK to write "I feel stuck" again and again until something else comes to mind. This exercise is essentially a brain drain. Write whatever comes to mind. Nothing is too silly or too stupid to be included. Do not read back what you have written for at least a few weeks.

Writing the morning pages is a great way to creative recovery!

2: The Pennebaker exercise

Is there something in your life that you are particularly worried or upset about right now? If it has been on your mind for some weeks, this is a technique that you might like to try. Commit to writing about the issue that is worrying you for at least 15 minutes a day for the next three or four days consecutively. The ideal time to do this is at the end of the day, and without interruption. Write about your problem from different perspectives; what is the problem? What is making you worried about it? What positives might there be in this situation? What might a friend or relative say to you if you told them about this situation? How could you look at it differently?

Write about the situation from as many different perspectives as you can. Writing your thoughts and feelings down about a specific issue really can help to analyse and change your feeling and approach to it.

3: The step back and ask why approach

This can be helpful in helping you to get over events in the past that are particularly upsetting.

Close your eyes and go back to the time of the experience and see the scene in your mind's eye. Now take a few steps back (in your mind). Move away from the situation to a point where you can now watch the event unfold from a distance and see yourself in the event. As you do this, focus on what has now become distant to you. Now watch the experience unfold as if it were happening to the distant you all over again. Take a few moments to replay the event as it unfolds in your imagination and to observe your distant self.

Continue to watch the situation unfold to your distant self, and as you do so seek to understand her/his feelings. Ask yourself what are the underlying causes and reasons for this situation?

Sue Williams is a poet, author and creator of the award-winning Believe Oracle Cards app. She achieved best-seller status in her category on Amazon for *"I Am Unique"* her first poetry book. Two further anthologies in the Believe series: *"Believe You Can Face Your Fears and Confidently Claim the Life You Desire* and *Believe You Can Live a Life You Love at 50+* are available on Amazon.

You can find Sue at www.sue-williams.com

THE JOURNEY
Sue Williams

Now that I know, dare I let it all go?
Tear up that script, that screed,
prevention to succeed?
Let it drift downstream, get lost in the surf;
Turf out old dreams; sometimes screams,
from long ago:
The nightmares they became.

Allow myself to ease into my flow, really let go?
The twists, the turns that led me here,
suddenly became a map, so clear;
Of yesterday's roads, no longer to be travelled;
Now, helped; unravelled,
What if I take one step, make one choice?
State in my OWN voice,
That I choose a different path?
Once again, renewed;
Begin to feel.
Allow my aching heart,
unhesitatingly, to heal.

THIS IS ME!
~ *Jackie Wilson*

"How does one become a butterfly?" Pooh asked pensively. "You must want to fly so much that you are willing to give up being a caterpillar," Piglet replied. A.A. Milne

I'm a shy 13-year-old girl sitting in class, when the teacher asks a question. As is often the case, I know the answer and yet cannot bring myself to put my hand up. If I do and I'm chosen, I will go bright red, and feel really embarrassed when everyone is looking at me. "Oh no." I'm chosen anyway! Sick with embarrassment, I wish I could just disappear. I feel ugly. I see so many beautiful girls and I'm not one of them. I just want to hide away. I feel so angry at the world; I don't fit in, I'm a bad person.

Fast forward. I'm 45 years old, married to an amazing man, with three beautiful children. I am an author, a keynote speaker and radio presenter who has created self-empowerment programmes. I deliver these to children, teens, young adults, parents and educators to help them to grow in self-awareness, mindset, self-belief, resilience and to achieve their potential.

How did I achieve such a transformation? I truly feel that it has so much to do with the word BELIEVE. Look in the middle of the word and you will see the word LIE.

I had created so many beliefs that I thought were true during my childhood, you may relate to some of them –

"I am ugly", "I'm not good enough", "I'm not loved" or "I'm not important" and so many more.

When I was three years old my little sister was born, and I realise now it was from that moment that I created limiting beliefs such as "I'm not important", "I'm not loved", and "I'm not good enough". Time and time again people told me I was a shy kid, and I completely believed the label.

My uncle, who I was very close to, died in a tragic accident when I was 10 years old. I had no support system during that time as my parents were suffering and focused on supporting my grandparents at the same time.

No-one was to blame; it was just overlooked that I also needed support. Although I have no memory of the time after my uncle passed due to shock, I realised I suppressed my grief to protect Mum from further stress.

Unfortunately, if grief is not dealt with, it will find a way out through another channel and, for me as a teen, that came physically by creating a skin reaction of dermatitis, along with anger. I became a very angry teen, and another belief was set that I was a bad person. I hated myself, hated my body, hated who I was (who I thought I was).

Over the years, the dermatitis became less, but the anger stayed. I met my now-husband at the age of 17. We were friends for two years, and we became a couple when I was 19, and at 23, we had our first daughter. Our son followed nearly two years later. Unfortunately, that was a difficult time for me as my limiting beliefs played out in my relationship; my anger was shared between my husband and my children. Being a parent is probably one of the most challenging experiences we can have, especially when coupled with poor mental health, and no self-awareness. I felt so low. I was continuously enraged; I felt like a failure as a parent, but on the outside to friends, family and people I came into contact with, I showed little signs of suffering.

My first step into the holistic world came with attending yoga sessions, which I really connected with. These brought moments of peace, and time for me. It created some relief from my poor mental health, as I reflect back. I always left a class feeling uplifted; the calm and space practising yoga created in my mind, and the physical shifts in my body were crucial in my journey.

My son suffered with eczema from a baby, and I wasn't keen on putting chemicals on his little body. I happened to come across a book called *What Really Works for Kids* which led me to investigate alternative natural treatment, and from that moment, I have been engrossed in learning about healing the body and mind.

In that book, I came across a section on yoga for children. My daughter used to join me in doing yoga, and what caught my eye was how yoga poses had been renamed to relate to the imagination of kids – the dog, the candle, the cat. That got my attention. I wondered if

268

there were classes for children, and searched the internet but couldn't find any. Soon, an idea sprang to mind. I could train to be a children's yoga teacher! I began searching, but couldn't find any training at all. Six months later, the idea just hadn't gone away, so I looked again and, discovering a course, booked myself on.

Employed by a tour operator as a travel consultant, things had reached a point where office work wasn't working out for me. So, in June 2003 I set off on my new adventure as a kids' yoga teacher.

That wasn't easy for me. I still carried very limiting beliefs about myself and my abilities, and I really had to force myself to sit in front of my daughter's class with a teacher and run my first session. Goodness, I was so nervous and terrified, having 30 faces looking expectantly up at me! However, a little spark of courage inside drove me forwards through the challenge.

I then set up after school clubs at the school, and ran classes in the community, and became very busy working in schools and day nurseries. I discovered that I loved working with children. I didn't feel judged, rather, I felt accepted. Those old, negative beliefs only popped up when I had difficult children and every time I would fall back into my 'I'm not good enough' mantra.

My mental health was still a struggle. Teaching yoga was an escape from my reality, and I did further training to develop my yoga for older children, teens and a two-year adult teacher training course. I absolutely thrived on teaching. However, my lack of self-worth returned once I stepped back into everyday life. Whilst away with friends one weekend, I reached the peak of my negative emotional state. My friend faced me with some truths about myself and I broke down. The self-hatred was spoken about for the first time, and I cried and cried. I felt broken; I had had enough of myself.

So, I went to see a doctor, who advised me I was depressed. This wasn't a label I accepted, and I refused medication, but did take up the option of going for counselling. My marriage was at rock bottom, my life was a mess. For a few weeks I went to see both a counsellor and a marriage counsellor.

Life began to improve a little. Having experienced how counselling helped me, I found an evening course on first level counselling and enrolled. Although I completed the course, it didn't feel right for me to become a counsellor. I also discovered Reiki and became attuned to levels 1 and 2, and for a time, I worked with clients. From this point on I knew that I wanted to continue learning about natural healing.

Many years later, life was still a challenge, yet improving all of the time. A friend asked if I wanted to be part of a year-long pilot programme in self-development. I jumped at the chance! Four of us embarked on a journey which would turn my life completely around. On this programme I experienced the feeling of waking up to reality, recognising how I was affecting my life, the dramas I created, the passing down of generations of beliefs, and so much more. I reflected on why I did the job I did, realising I was projecting my lack of self-belief onto the kids; I was teaching by using particular positive affirmations. In an emotional moment of clarity, I realised these were what I myself needed to embody!

Through participating in this programme, I felt that I had woken up to life. I discovered that life didn't have to happen to me, life could happen for me; I just needed to create awareness and notice what I was doing. Towards the end of the programme we were also guided to discover our purpose. Mine is to educate the next generation with knowledge of who they really are, to empower them to be able to navigate life more easily and to be their potential.

My lasting memory of that programme is of sitting in the garden on a late summer day and being asked to choose an emblem to symbolise our journey. For me it was a butterfly, because I had felt like a caterpillar just moving through life, and I had no idea that I had always had wings and the ability to fly. Just at that moment a butterfly landed on my shoulder – coincidence or synchronicity? I choose to believe the latter.

Since completing that programme, I have chosen to allow life to happen for me. Gradually, I began piecing my jigsaw of life together, becoming more self-aware, noticing when I had fallen back into my old story and my

271

negative beliefs, and starting to make changes. I have used my inner resources such as courage, determination, and passion to step up by facing my fears around public speaking, going on radio and TV, delivering programmes to adults (yes that was a fear), writing a book and more.

I continue my professional development to enhance the work I do with the next generation and the ecosystem around them. I believe that everyone has the ability to have successful and fulfilling lives, no matter your background, race, gender, or academic ability.

For me, it's all down to mindset, having self-belief and determination to be more than you believe you can be. Every day I continue to raise the bar for myself, to be a role model for my own children and all the children I have the pleasure of working with. I'm in a place now where I have changed my belief system to be able to say "I love and accept myself for all that I am – This is ME!"

I currently work in schools and the community with children, parents and educators, taking them on a journey of self-discovery so they can find their 'treasure' within, find their greatness, the truth of who they are. When we accept our uniqueness, see our brilliance, and have a 'toolkit' to support us to navigate life's challenges, we are more able to be our potential, be compassionate and empathic to the difficulties others face, and step forward into a successful and fulfilling life.

If you want to improve your self-belief, my tips to you are:

1: Create an awareness of your inner critic, that little voice that criticises you. Mindfulness is a great way to notice that voice and observe it without being attached to it.

2: Realise that happiness is inside us, covered in layers of self-doubt, frustration, anger at the world that gives us the message that happiness is found if we have an amazing body, we are beautiful, have wealth and material things. I have learnt this is not true.

3: Start looking for your 'inner treasure chest'. Within it are your qualities, attributes and strengths, a place where you can discover your inner greatness and that YOU ARE ENOUGH'. You are an amazing, unique, important and extraordinary person who deserves a wonderful life and to achieve your potential.

Jackie Wilson is a Self-Development and Emotional Well-Being Specialist, providing emotional resilience and self-development training in schools and organisations. She is the Founder of both Empower Education and The Well-Being Hub for Families and Schools. She is also Author of the upcoming book – *This is ME!* written for teens, and Co-Author of "The Book of Inspiration for Women by Women."
www.empowereducation.co.uk

YOUR LEGACY
Sue Williams

If you were to utter a small word
At the end of the world,
What would it be?
Would it be "pride", or "joy" or "pain",
What sense, from living, did you garner or gain?

A sense of true purpose; heartfelt belief,
A shining example; or filled with misgivings,
guilt and grief?
Radiating "fun", perhaps joie de vivre,
Or down-trodden with "dread";
dismayed, take your leave?

Words have real meaning; powerful, vibrant and strong,
Would you choose one that questions:
Did you truly belong?
Feeling "alone"; drab and distant; duly depart,
Not able to speak with real "love", from the heart?

I urge you; banish "doubt", "mistrust" and "fear"
What need for such bleak, worrisome words to appear?
When there is "awe", "wonder", "magic"; a "gift"
Words that sad, sorry spirits of others,
so surely would lift?

Take "vim", "verve" and "vision" with you when you go,
For in reality, you truly don't know,
Whether your one, small word might plant a seed,
That a magnificent, new;
yet still imperfect, world may come to need!

ABOUT THE AUTHOR

Aged 51, Sue Williams took early retirement from her career with the Civil Service, having worked in career information, advice and guidance services for adults for over 21 years. Her own early career aspirations were thwarted when she felt too lacking in confidence to explore a career in journalism during her late teens. Unsure of what else to do, she initially took a teacher training course, and later retrained, achieving a Postgraduate Diploma in Careers Guidance in 1991.

On leaving employment, Sue embarked on a journey of exploration, which resulted in a new career in writing and publishing. She started journaling each morning, which unexpectedly led to her writing in rhyme!

She has now published and is lead author in three anthologies of true stories aimed at inspiring women to have more self-belief and confidence; *Believe You Can, Believe You Can Succeed,* and *Believe You Can Live a Life You Love at 50+.* She achieved No.1 status in her category on Amazon for her first collection of poetry; *I Am Unique* and also achieved a Janey Loves Gold award for her inspirational Believe Oracle cards app in 2017.

Sue has run events for authors, including her first major national event "*Your Signature Success Story*", in 2016.

For more information, please go to Sue's website:

www.sue-williams.com.

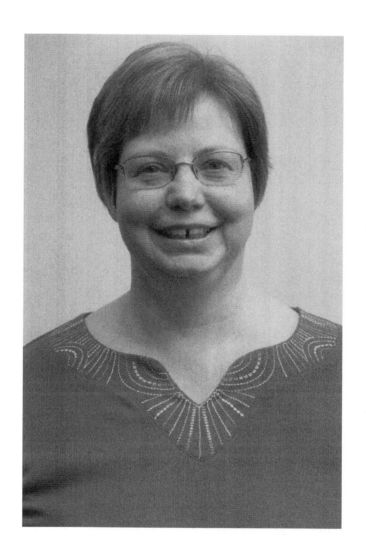

ADDITIONAL PRODUCTS & SERVICES

The *Believe You Can Journal*

With so many exercises, hints and tips to try, it is a great idea to have a copy of the *Believe You Can Journal* to hand. Use it to jot down any thoughts, questions and feelings that arise as you do the exercises. You might also write out affirmations or actions that you want to use or take. You may even want to compose a poem, or do some doodling to get your creative juices flowing. It will form a record of your growing self-belief and where that self-nurturing has taken you.

Believe You Can Face Your Fears and Confidently Claim the Life You Desire and *Believe You Can Live a Life You Love at 50+.*

Two further collections of true stories and poems for women on the topic of self-belief.

Both available to purchase on Amazon.

The Believe Oracle Cards app

Believe Oracle Cards are a simple and effective way of getting to know yourself and learning how to overcome challenges you face. These uplifting cards were created to give you a quick boost each day. Choose a card at random to receive a short, inspirational message to reflect on, and to encourage you to take action.

For further details see www.sue-williams.com

GRATITUDE

Thank you for having the belief to read this book.

If you have enjoyed reading it,

and would like to help others

to share the inspiration in the uplifting stories,

please take a few moments

to leave your honest review on Amazon.

Sue Williams
www.sue-williams.com

Printed in Poland
by Amazon Fulfillment
Poland Sp. z o.o., Wrocław

54205400R00163